The Genius of
Natural Childhood

The Genius of Natural Childhood

Secrets of Thriving Children

SALLY GODDARD BLYTHE

Contributors

JANE WILLIAMS, PETER BLYTHE
AND ARLETTE OVERMAN

Illustrations by

SHARON RENTTA
AND
TOM KERR

The Genius of Natural Childhood © 2011 Sally Goddard Blythe

Sally Goddard Blythe is hereby identified as the author of this work in accordance with section 77 of the Copyright, Designs and Patent Act, 1988. She asserts and gives notice of her moral right under this Act.

Published by Hawthorn Press, Hawthorn House,
1 Lansdown Lane, Stroud, Gloucestershire, GL5 1BJ, UK
Tel: (01453) 757040   Fax: (01453) 751138
E-mail: info@hawthornpress.com
Website: www.hawthornpress.com

Cover illustration © Getty Images
Cover design by Lucy Guenot, Bookcraft Ltd
Illustrations by Sharon Rentta and Tom Kerr
Typesetting by Bookcraft Ltd, Stroud, Glos GL5 1AA
Printed by Henry Ling Ltd, The Dorset Press, Dorchester

Every effort has been made to trace the ownership of all copyrighted material. If any omission has been made, please bring this to the publisher's attention so that proper acknowledgement may be given in future editions.

Printed on paper sourced from sustained managed forests and elemental chlorine free

British Library Cataloguing in Publication Data applied for

ISBN 978-1-907359-04-0

For Henry Alexander,
the first of my grandchildren,
and
my other grandchildren waiting to be.

Contents

Acknowledgements

I am indebted to:

Martin Large, who first suggested this book several years before I was ready to write it, and continued to prompt me every few months to consider turning his idea into reality. His faith in my ability, his patience with my procrastinations, and his suggestions and support throughout the writing of the book have been invaluable.

Jane Williams PhD, Director of Toddler Kindy GymbaROO in Australia for writing Chapter 4 and sharing ideas and activities from the Toddler Kindy GymbaROO programme.

Tom Kerr for the illustrations accompanying Chapter 4.

Professor Yair Schiftan for his wisdom, experience and sharing of knowledge about the importance of vibration for life, development and healing.

Professor Michael Lazarev for his insight and enthusiasm in explaining the science behind early communication, for providing a medical and pedagogic structure for mother-infant interaction, for marrying the artistic and scientific disciplines of music and medicine, and most of all for his poetry and music, which have benefited many thousands of children not only in Russia but increasingly in the rest of the world.

Arlette Overman for her contribution, 'A music teacher's perspective on the importance of music in the early years' in Chapter 2.

Dr. Peter Blythe for rewriting *When two hearts were one*, a fairy story for adults, originally written when he was a young man returning home from the Far East at the end of the Second World War.

Sharon Rentta for her timeless illustrations to accompany the chapters on lullabies, nursery rhymes and 'A Day in the Garden', and for the CD *Wings of Childhood*.

Roque and his parents for recording and sharing images of the first year of his life.

Charlotte, Maisie, Annabel, Zoe and their parents for sharing and giving permission for pictures of their natural childhood to be included.

Eve and her parents for making available photographs of exercise positions for Chapter 6.

Amanda Engelbach, editor of *The Montessori European Journal*, for permission to use an excerpt from the article 'Why boys and girls needs are different in the early years', originally published in *The Montessori European Journal*, April–June 2010.

The Community Care Inform website for allowing me to rework material originally written for them.

My editor Matthew Barton, who pointed out where sections needed modifying, corrected my mistakes, suggested additions, improved my wording, and made this book more readable.

And all who have been involved in the production of this book at Hawthorn Press.

Foreword

RICHARD HOUSE, PH.D.
ROEHAMPTON UNIVERSITY

Did many pre-technological ways of raising children often get it right after all? In her eagerly awaited new book, Sally Goddard-Blythe allies the virtues of 'old-fashioned' music and movement with the latest insights of neuroscience, to demonstrate just this. *The Genius of Natural Childhood* is tailor-written for a technology-saturated generation of young parents who (through no fault of their own) are increasingly losing the capacity to live playfully and 'just be' with their young children. For this reason alone, this book should find its way onto the bookshelf of every enlightened parent and education professional.

I first came across Sally's ground-breaking work over a decade ago when training in early-childhood (Steiner) education; and several years later, as the then editor of Hawthorn Press's innovative *Early Years* series (to which this book is the latest addition), I was delighted to help commission her seminal book, *The Well Balanced Child: Movement and Early Learning* (2nd edition, 2005). Sally's work is an inspiration to all who believe that young children's developmental journeys are best understood and supported through genuinely holistic perspectives. More specifically, in showing us why *the body* needs to be at the centre of early child development, Sally follows in the auspicious footsteps of some of our greatest philosophers and theorists of early learning, not least Maurice Merleau-Ponty, Rudolf Steiner and Donald Winnicott. Winnicott, for one, would surely turn in his grave if he could witness the overly cognitive, body-neglecting, early-learning 'regimes' to which a new generation of youngsters is often subjected – and which, incredibly, is increasingly dictated by state regulations.

I write regularly for *The Mother* magazine, and a young parent recently wrote this in response to one of my articles:

> The bit about how all parents and early years workers should be trained **not** to intervene in the young child's 'going-on being' [really struck me] ... I was a very 'conscientious' first-time mother, wanting to accelerate my daughter's learning experience in every way possible. This involved structuring her day around what I thought she needed ... – [but] I always found [this approach] instinctively wrong, too fast-paced for a small child, and exhausting for me! I used to feel I was being somehow neglectful if I wasn't 'doing' something with my child. Thankfully, when my daughter turned two, I ... discovered a wonderful local Steiner Waldorf school ... [When she first visited the nursery there] ... it felt so right, and it felt like coming home. My daughter has thrived there ever since in the calm, harmonious and gentle environment ... I am much happier, more positive/ contented and couldn't now give two hoots about whether my daughter has reached all the right milestones ... As I am now close to welcoming our second child ... I want to offer space, comfort and love rather than 'early educational experiences'... I keep myself ... occupied with my own useful activities (writing, painting, household chores, gardening, baking) rather than focusing all of my energies on my child. She happily imitates my activity one minute and then runs off for hours to play on her own without any need for me to disturb her. Less is definitely more ...

This letter comes from a parent struggling with the challenges of parenting today in our technological and often hyperactive age. It is a moving testimony that, in my view, is worth more than all the words of a hundred childcare or child-development 'experts'. The more such experts dispense their advice to parents, the more parents may believe that they *need* such expertise to fulfil their parenting role effectively – a self-fulfilling prophecy (as the late, great Ivan Illich pointed out many years ago).

It is notoriously difficult for professionals to relinquish their advice-giving identity, and focus instead on empowering parents to find *their own* path of relating to their new baby or young child. I raise this issue of 'over-professionalised' expertise because the approach adopted in this book offers parents a way out of this disempowering cul-de-sac. It reaffirms, instead, perennial wisdom and child-friendly practices that are in great danger of being lost in our modern(ist) techno-culture. Sally's work therefore falls squarely in the tradition of the great paediatrician Donald Winnicott who, many decades ago, wrote and spoke with wonderful eloquence about the innate wisdom that parents have in parenting their own children.

So, welcome to a magical treasure-house, and to the genius of holistic early development and learning. I strongly commend this book to you, parent and practitioner alike; and if only early years teacher training courses would embrace the simple yet profound thinking that is present here in abundance, the well-being of young children everywhere would be vitally enhanced.

Dr Richard House
Research Centre for Therapeutic Education
Roehampton University
London, April 2011

Introduction

With so much emphasis on getting children ready for reading, writing and numeracy in the early years, it is important to remember that the ability to understand and use written language and to fit in with others socially is built upon earlier physical foundations which are developed in the early (pre-school) years. Physical interaction with the environment and social engagement with parents and family are two of the vital ingredients for later social integration and educational achievement.

Forty years ago, the family was primarily responsible for the process of 'bringing up' children, or educating them in the general sense, with school providing specific instruction in literacy, numeracy and academic subjects. Today, by contrast, we are increasingly witnessing a growing dependence on school and state to provide and nurture all aspects of children's growth and education. For many families, shared time and activities are increasingly rare, and the state emphasizes getting mothers and fathers back to work. Rather than supporting childcare at home, it focuses increasingly on early years nursery provision.

Since the dawn of the new millennium, daily reports in the media have highlighted such problems as poor literacy standards in schools; children starting school unable to manage simple motor tasks (such as the ability to use a knife and fork); poor listening skills; poor attention; increase in childhood obesity; children of working mothers having unhealthier lifestyles; increase in autistic-type behaviours; and children entering school with immature speech and language. There have been several reports that around 40 per cent of parents admit they *never* read to their child; and that a new generation of parents across the social spectrum are, for a variety of reasons, unaware of the importance of physical development and the role of movement, music and interactive play in the early years for building the foundations for later learning.

Since the 1950s, society has undergone a technological revolution, with sweeping changes to lifestyle as radical as the agricultural and industrial revolutions of the seventeenth to nineteenth centuries. This technological revolution has also brought about an increase in the *speed* of change, which now occurs at such a rapid rate that we are frequently oblivious of what is being lost, as well as gained, in the relentless pursuit of progress. The real impact of rapid environmental change on human development will only be known in the future, but we are already witnessing the effects of sedentary lifestyles and changes in the working lives of parents on children's development. In a debate at Roehampton Institute of Education, author and professor of journalism Rosalind Coward said:

> Many would scoff at the suggestion that modern society is bad for children. Of course it isn't they say. Look at infant mortality figures. Look at general health and longevity. Look at our welfare system – a net to protect children from absolute poverty. Or the fact all children have the right to education. Modern society allows children not only to survive but to expect a reasonably fulfilled adult life. In comparison to the past, or less affluent societies, our children are remarkably privileged. Yet evidence is mounting that these privileges have not brought contentment. Ever younger children are exhibiting symptoms of mental illness: self-harming, eating disorders, and disturbed or aggressive behaviour. The adults they become are also more stressed and less happy than many apparently less privileged societies. Psychologist Oliver James calls it 'affluenza'.[1]

During the same debate, educationalist Richard House said:

> The medicalization of children's experience, and high-stakes testing and managerialist 'audit culture' values have swamped educational experience and deprived children of their birthright – the right to enjoy and be empowered by a developmentally appropriate learning environment. I believe that the various 'symptoms' of distress we have labelled 'toxic childhood' should

be interpreted as children's insightful commentary on just how badly we adults are doing, rather than some 'psychopathology' that needs to be medicalized and 'treated'.[2]

Most people would accept that children thrive when they are nurtured by committed parents in the context of a close-knit family and community. Modern lifestyles have done much to destroy this primary nurturing environment.

These factors, combined with the loss of traditional rhymes, stories and games from children's experience, and parents' knowledge, mean that parents increasingly do not know what to do or *why* traditional games were important for children's development. Parents are asking such things as: What can we do to help our child's development? How can we prevent our child from having reading problems, or being labelled with a specific learning difficulty like attention deficit disorder (ADD)? Why are teachers complaining about our child's behaviour? Parents are often misled into believing that more cognitive stimulation in the form of the teaching of formal skills from an early age, extra-curricular activities or electronic games provide the answer. While each of these can help with specific problems, parents and early years educators need to be aware of the broader context of children's development and to know *why* physical development through play, in the context of involvement with close family members in the early years, is an essential precursor to later educational success and emotional wellbeing.

A plethora of advice is available for those who seek it on how to bring up children, how to get your child to sleep and to eat, how to deal with tantrums, etc, but much less on what *children* really need, or information on how long-held traditions supported healthy child development in the past. While social structures and lifestyles have changed at breakneck speed since the fifties, the developmental needs of children remain much the same. An increasing percentage of parents in the modern technological world have themselves had no experience of being parented by a full-time parent, and consequently may be unaware of the benefits of this. Many do not know how to provide materials and activities to keep their children amused or why the simpler lives of previous generations may have produced better educated and more socially sympathetic individuals. This book aims to provide a 'starter pack' for such parents on both why and how everything a child needs can be drawn from the fundamentals of life available to everyone – beginning with the importance of movement and sensory experience in the early years.

Rather than developing yet another 'new programme', the book offers examples of traditional lullabies, nursery rhymes, stories and games, and explains how they actually develop children's skills at different ages and stages of development. In this way parents can revive and enjoy with their children the songs, stories and games of past generations, and adapt them to modern needs.

As an example of how stories, for instance, can feed directly into enlivening play, Chapter 6 introduces a story, 'A Day in the Garden'. The story comprises a series of animal characters whose movement characteristics loosely mirror important periods of physical development from infancy to age five. Parents are encouraged to read the story to their children, familiarize them with the characters and then encourage children to 'act out' the story in physical play.

Chapter 7 discusses the issue of physical 'readiness' for school, providing suggestions for developing school readiness, what to look out for in a child who is not quite 'ready' for school, and which agencies may be able to help.

How to use this book

Chapters 1, 2 and 7 explain *why* certain activities support development, while chapters 3, 4 and 6 provide examples of activities which translate such theory into practice, showing *how* one can support children's development.

Chapter 5 explores the importance and significance of fairy tales, fables and bedtime stories in the modern world.

The reader is invited to go straight to chapters which seem of immediate interest first. Young parents for example may prefer to start with the more practical 'how' chapters, while professionals involved in child development may prefer to begin with 'why'. It is hoped that if you begin with 'how' chapters you will eventually want to return to explore 'why' many of the traditions, lullabies, nursery rhymes, games and stories of the past remain essential for children today, to pass them on to your children so that when they become parents, they will instinctively pass them on to theirs. In this way, every parent becomes a custodian of the language, literature, music and general culture from which he* grew.

Notes

1 R. Coward: 'Is modern society bad for children?' debate at Roehampton University, available online at http://www.theinstituteofwellbeing.com/blog/?p=433&cpage=1. 2009
2 Ibid.

---

* To avoid the awkward use of both genders, I will alternate from chapter to chapter

CHAPTER I

Movement – The Expression of Life

Movement as language

Movement is the very expression of life. Long before a child develops spoken language, her feelings and thoughts come to spontaneous expression through the medium of movement – which is therefore her very first language. Young children jump for joy, shrink back in fear, or reach out in anticipation. Adults, so often constrained or comparatively inexpressive in their own bodies, easily understand what these childish movements mean. Conversely, when adults exaggerate their gestures and movements, as clowns do, children immediately understand the emotions they convey.

The late Professor E. J. Kiphard, known to many as the 'father of motorology' in Germany, provided a personal illustration of how the language of movement and mime communicates at all levels. Professor Kiphard was Chair of Preventative Treatment and Rehabilitation through Exercise and Sport at the Sports Institute in Frankfurt. He was also E. J. Kiphard the clown, who visited centres for physically handicapped children, complete with bright red nose and bowler hat. One journalist reporting on his work described how

> ... children identify with this clumsy figure who combs his hair with a giant comb, makes water appear from fragments of paper, and who stumbles around in colossal boots frequently falling flat on his face. This adult clown, dressed in children's clothes, seemingly more helpless than they themselves, becomes an

approachable character; the children come out of themselves and take on responsibilities. An autistic child reacted unexpectedly to an especially awkward act, exclaiming, 'I want to help you, you poor old silly clown.' It was because of such results that Professor Kiphard was convinced that adults should 'clown more often'.[1]

Body language is not only an essential part of communication; its development precedes spoken language. When a child's movement vocabulary is well-developed, she is better able not only to express herself through non-verbal means but also to understand the body language of others. This is the beginning of empathy (which literally means 'feeling what another feels').

Even after speech has developed, if the right words cannot be found older children and adults will revert to the language of gesture as an alternative way of expressing themselves. Think, for example, of what it is like as an adult trying to order from a menu or explain what is wrong with your car in a foreign country where you do not speak the language. Gesticulation then becomes the basic form of communication (one of the reasons why the telephone is no help!). An upset child will naturally withdraw eye contact, cling to her mother, or kick and scream. This is communication at its most basic level – behaviour – and although we may not understand the reasons for the distress unless we have witnessed the events leading up to it (context), distress expressed through the medium of posture and gesture can be universally understood.

Babies are born mimics. In the 1970s and 80s a group of scientists carried out studies in which they observed mother and infant inter-actions.[2] They noticed that babies will imitate simple adult gestures, such as sticking out the tongue, soon after birth. This early capacity to imitate the movements, facial expressions and gestures of others is part of a 'mirror neuron' system, which is able to sense, recognize and reproduce the mannerisms of other people.[3] A few years later it was discovered that mirror neurons do indeed exist in a part of the brain called the pre-motor cortex.*

---

* When investigated in macaque monkeys, mirror neurons fired not only when a monkey performed an action itself, but also when it observed another living creature perform the same action. (Gallese V, Fadiga I and Rizzolatti G, 1996: 'Action recognition in the pre-motor cortex'. *Brain* 119: 593–609). A theory

The implications of these findings for child development are that infants need *interactive communication,* where they can both observe *and* imitate the movements, gestures and expressions of others in order to assimilate them and develop a non-verbal vocabulary of their own. The non-verbal elements of language are believed to contribute up to 90 per cent of effective communication.

Activity is the natural expression of the waking state, never more so than in the early years of life when understanding of the world is acquired through *interaction* with people and the environment – physically through movement experience and contact, socially through *interaction and engagement* with other human beings, and emotionally through a combination of these.

Learning through movement

When a baby is born she has minimal voluntary control over her bodily movements, which come in bursts of energy with little conscious regulation of force or speed. A baby's efforts to touch or grasp repeatedly overshoot or miss their target, but gradually over the first months of life these movements become more refined.

At first a baby does not understand that her hands and feet are part of her own body: they are simply objects or playthings which randomly come and go from her field of vision. She does not yet 'know' that the position of her hands may be determined by where her head is, simply following her hand movements with her eyes. This is because an infant reflex ties head, arm and eye movements together. Movement of the hand away from the face helps to extend visual focusing distance from near point (babies are shortsighted for the first few weeks of life) to arm's length; in this way movement or action

---

developed that by simulating action even when watching an act, the neurons allow us to recognize and understand other people's actions and intentions. This theory has been called into question by more recent research at Harvard University, which found evidence to suggest that when these neurons encounter repeated stimulus they reduce their successive response, a process called adaptation. If mirror neurons existed in the activated part of the brain, reasoned one of the researchers, adaptation should be triggered by both observation *and* performance. (Caramazza A.: *Proceedings of the National Academics of Science* [DOI: 10.1073/pnas.0902262106]. Cited in: P. Shetty. 'Role of the mirror neurons may need a rethink.' *New Scientist Life* 27/10, May 2009).

acts as the primary medium through which the sensory systems are entrained and learn how to work together in the first months of life. It will take many years of movement-guided, multi-sensory experience and integration to develop an adult sense of perception.

Similarly, when a baby kicks her legs, and succeeds in grasping her toes, she learns through feedback from the muscles, tendons and joints of the body, combined with vision and touch, where her body begins and ends in space.

Confidence in space also provides the physical basis for the growing sense of self. In the 1960s Ray Barsch described the young child as being a 'terranaut', an astronaut or explorer of space on terra firma. While the exploration of outer space may be one of the miracles of modern science, 'they are surpassed by the daily miracle of the newborn infant's conquest of terrestrial space'.[4] In this sense, every infant is a 'space pioneer' who must acquire spatial proficiency in the use of her own body to provide a firm foundation for life and learning.

Prenatal movement experience

During life inside the womb, the developing baby was able to sense every movement her mother made, but the type of movement she experienced was very different from movement as we come to know it after birth. This is because in the enclosed world of the womb she was surrounded by fluid and cushioned from the full force of gravity by the support provided by the mother's body, yet was still capable of sensing changes in the mother's position and the quality of her movements.

She was also able to make movements of her own, both in response to changes in her protected environment and as a fundamental expression of her developing nervous system:

> The prenate communicates its experiences the only way it can: through motility. Eye movement, heart-rate, respiration, gestures, and elimination patterns speak volumes about the individual prenatal world. The patterns that these expressions make, when attended to, add texture to our understanding of the quality of prenatal life. They also give us our first insights into who the unique being is within its mother's body. Prenatal movement patterns are replicated in the newborn, demonstrating the continuity of neural

behavior. The human fetus sleeps, breathes moves, eliminates, and feels, sees, cries, initiates and responds. He or she is acutely sensitive, as a result of constantly expanding neurological capacities, to the surrounding. This primary neurological unfolding is nourished and enhanced by parental awareness, dialogue and subtle touch on the mother's body which communicates directly with the baby.[5]

In the first few weeks after birth – far more than all the inventions designed to make parenthood easier – the comfort, reassurance and movement experience derived from being in close physical proximity to another human being, particularly the mother, replicate many of the movement experiences familiar from before birth. Adults naturally tend to rock, sway and carry a baby in order to soothe it, thereby simulating the movements which the baby experienced in the womb.

Physical contact

For centuries, mothers all over the world have carried their babies in their arms, in a sling, on their side or back. In many countries, Africa, India for example, and in tribal communities, this has developed for practical reasons as well as being a cultural habit that continues because it allows the parent to have free use of their hands to continue with daily chores, while remaining close to the baby.

In Asia and Africa, babies are carried by the mother, usually, in communities where farming and agriculture are very important. Mothers are thus able to tend to their daily activities with a baby strapped on their back, continuing for several months the dyadic relationship which was present between mother and baby before birth.[6]

What does baby carrying do?

- Baby carrying gives the baby a sense of closeness, safety and security through direct physical communication between mother (or carrier) and baby. This enables the carrier to pick up small changes in the baby's mood and respond. In certain cultures, mother and baby are so attuned to each other's bodily changes that western inventions such as nappies are not necessary. When a mother senses her baby needs to urinate or defecate – she simply lifts her away from her body and holds her over the ground.[7]

- The gentle motion provided by the mother's movements is comforting, providing constant and gentle stimulation to the balance mechanism. This provides a continuum from pre-natal to post-natal life at a time when the infant has minimal conscious control over her own movements.
- Baby carrying allows the carrier to 'tune in' to the baby's needs before she starts crying. As the mother becomes attuned to small changes in her baby's movements, levels of arousal, gestures and sounds, she is better able to respond immediately. This builds trust as well as confidence in the care-giver and security in the baby, and reduces the duration of fretting.
- One of the mother's roles has been described as acting as the baby's auxilliary cortex* or the external regulator of arousal and emotional state *before* the baby is able to do it for herself.[8] When mother and baby are in close proximity and attuned to each other's needs, mother can quickly respond to her baby, thus reducing anxiety. The baby can also start to learn to regulate basic needs such as hunger and comfort for herself, by having free access to the breast. This is just the beginning of being able to self-regulate levels of arousal and anxiety
- Baby carrying allows babies to share in the everyday movements and routine of their parent – walking, talking, laughing, movement and working. This creates an atmosphere of ongoing, daily learning, biological rhythm and social communication.

Training the senses through movement

Balance

Most people are familiar with the five senses of touch, taste, smell, vision and hearing. These are **external** senses, which provide information about stimuli received from outside the body; but we also have **internal** senses: of balance and proprioception (feedback derived

---

* Cerebral cortex – the part of the brain where billions of neurons work together to allow for consciousness and thought, movement and sensation, cognition and language, and other important tasks including, ultimately, the ability to regulate one's own emotions.

from the muscles, tendons and joints), which inform us about our position in space.

Each of the senses comprises specialized receptors sensitive to a specific range of movement frequencies (speed of motion). The balance mechanism for example responds particularly to slow, turning (rotation) or tilting movements and to movement that follows a linear direction (up and down or forward and back). The balance mechanism is most sensitive when movement starts, stops or when there is a variation in speed or direction.

The sense of touch responds to pressure or movement across the surface of the skin. These movements are generally faster than the type of movements detected by balance but not as fast as movements or vibrations sensed by hearing or vision.

Human hearing is able to detect vibrations travelling at speeds covering a range as wide as 20–20,000 hz* in the first weeks after birth. These different frequencies of vibration are perceived as pitch. This range of sound frequencies encompasses the sounds used in every human language, which is one reason why a baby, with adequate hearing, has the capacity to learn any language under the sun if exposed to the sounds of that language on a daily basis in the first years of life. During the first three years of life, a baby will learn to 'tune in' to the specific sounds of the language(s) spoken around her, rather like tuning into a radio station, but as she becomes more attuned to the sounds specific to her mother tongue or the local language, the ability to hear sounds that are not in regular use starts to fall away. This is why it is so much harder to learn a new language and to speak without a trace of accent at an older age. We will examine the importance of hearing and listening further in Chapter 2 in the context of music, communication and language.

Finally, the sense of sight, upon which we have become increasingly reliant in the modern world, specializes in detecting photons and waves of light travelling at speeds faster than the speed of sound. In other words, at a very basic level, each of the senses is actually a system of specific motion detectors. There is also an overlap in the sensitivity of the different sensory systems whereby very low frequency sound may be sensed by touch receptors as vibration,

---

* Hz (abbreviation of hertz) = unit of frequency equal to one cycle per second.

vibration can affect the sense of balance, and balance can affect how vision functions etc.

The external senses of hearing and vision are interdependent with the functioning of the internal senses. Both types must learn to work together to provide the brain with coherent information about the environment. When there is functional discrepancy between these two types of sensory system, it can result in distorted perception and a range of physical and emotional symptoms. One example of disagreement or discrepancy in the synchrony of different systems is the experience of motion sickness, which occurs when the relationship between balance, proprioception and vision is disturbed as a result of a particular type of (usually unaccustomed) motion.

The importance of congruence in the functioning of external and internal sensory systems for stable perception is illustrated by a couple of everyday examples. Imagine taking a ride at the fair on a merry-go-round. Rotation of the carousel and the up-and-down movements of the horse provide stimulation to the balance mechanism in the inner ear. After stepping off the carousel, for a few moments it can feel as if the ground is moving under your feet and the outside world also seems to be moving. You might feel nauseous and momentarily disorientated. This is because the balance mechanism contains fluid, which is set in motion by rotation and the up-and-down motion of the carousel. If there has been continuous increased stimulation for a period of time, the fluid in the inner ear continues to move for a few moments longer when the movement stops. Because centres involved in vision also receive signals from the balance mechanism, the visual system is temporarily confused and the brain thinks the external world is moving.

A similar sensation can occur if you are sitting in a stationary train and a train alongside you starts to pull out of the station. The brain is momentarily fooled into thinking that your train is the one that is moving. This is because the visual stimulus reaches the brain before signals from the body which would normally accompany active movement, temporarily tricking the brain.

Internal and external senses learn to work together in perfect timing (integration) through movement experience, practice and repetition in many different positions, at different speeds and under varying conditions. This is why physical activity is an essential part of the learning process. Practice not only improves performance over time, but also reduces the amount of mental energy required to carry out the task, increasing flexibility of response and adaptability to changing conditions.

Balance is the first of the sensory systems to develop, being formed at just 8 weeks after conception, functioning at 16 weeks after conception and myelinated* at the time of birth in a baby born at full term. Early maturation of the balance system reflects the essential role that balance plays in enabling a child to function well in a gravity-based environment. Without balance it would not be possible to sit, crawl or stand; you would not be able to control the movements of your eyes or integrate information derived from the senses to form a coherent perception of the outside world. Although the balance system is formed and ready for use at birth, it will take a young child many years to learn how to *use* the system efficiently. Learning to use the balance mechanism is like being given a grand piano as a present. Unless the child learns how to *play* the piano, it will either stand silent or be strummed discordantly and will never yield its full range of possibilities.

Floor play – baby's first independent playground

Although babies thrive on close physical contact in the first months of life, they also enjoy moments of independent exploration and free movement, and the ground provides an ideal space for this.

The first postural skill a baby must learn is to support her head. Head control is important because the position of the head influences how other muscle groups operate further down the body. General development of posture and tone follow a head-to-toe and centre-outwards progression. As the infant's head is large and heavy compared with her body, and has only limited muscle tone, learning to support the head is a major challenge. Babies usually start to lift their head when lying on the tummy (prone position) from as early

---

*   Myelin is an electrically insulating material that forms a layer, the myelin sheath. Usually, myelin surrounds only the axon of a neuron. It is essential for proper functioning of the nervous system, enabling information to be efficiently transmitted.

4–6 weeks, but it will take many more months for other muscles to strengthen throughout the body.

A biological theory originating in the 1800s stated that ontogeny (the origin and development of an individual organism from embryo to adult) recapitulates phylogeny (the evolutionary history of the species).[9] This theory has long since been discounted in its literal sense, but in a functional sense every child retraces many of the evolutionary steps of her forebears in terms of the movement patterns she learns to make and stages of language development in the early years.[10]

In the first year of life, a baby runs through a fast forward 'replay' of her ancestral history in the type and range of movements she learns to make. Before birth, floating inside her tiny private ocean inside the womb, movements were fish-like and perfectly adapted for life in water, where the effects of gravity are reduced. After birth, a baby must quickly start to develop muscle tone in order to support her own body weight against gravity, and this control begins with control of the head. Movements in the first twelve months progress from kicking, punching, 'cycling', and reaching from a fixed position, to crawling on the belly (reptilian), crawling on hands and knees like a mammal, and briefly passing through a simian (ape-like) phase, when she can pull herself up to stand for a few moments but must still use hands and arms to aid balance. Only when a child is able to stand and walk unsupported and the hands are freed from involvement in posture and balance do the skills unique to the human race – such as spoken language, fine motor control and eventually the ability to understand and use written language – start to develop.

Why floor play?

The floor provides the perfect playground for a baby's developing postural abilities, and muscles are used and developed in different ways depending on whether the baby is placed to lie on her tummy (prone) or back (supine).

Lying on the back on a firm and safe surface, a baby is free to kick her legs, flex and stretch her toes, wave her arms and use her neck muscles to try to lift her head. Every one of these movements provides feedback to the brain about position in space whilst also developing muscle tone. Vision is also relatively unrestricted when lying on the back, enabling the baby to scan her surroundings, search, reach, stretch and grasp.

Figures 1.1–1.13 illustrate some of the range of movements available to an infant who is placed on the floor and allowed unrestricted movement. From the uncontrolled movements seen in figures 1.1–1.3 and the early reflex reaction seen in figure 1.4 (when the baby turns the head to one side, the arm and leg extend on the side to which the head is turned, and the opposite limbs flex) to being able to turn, reach, grasp and bring an object back to the midline shown in figures 1.5, 1.6, and 1.7. In the first months of life, the mouth is the main arena of discovery. Furnished with millions of neural connections, before control of posture and hand-eye coordination have advanced, a baby uses her mouth to explore shape, size and texture. This involves being able to bring the hands to the midline as shown in figures 1.7, 1.8 and 1.9.

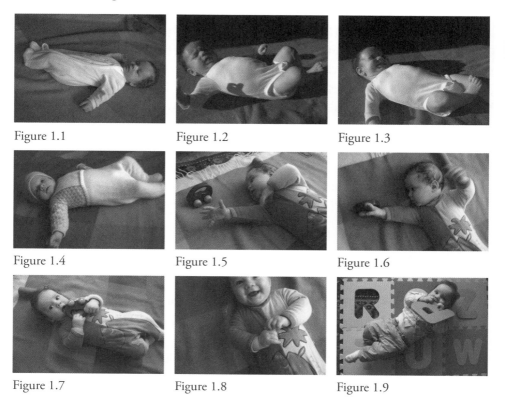

Figure 1.1   Figure 1.2   Figure 1.3

Figure 1.4   Figure 1.5   Figure 1.6

Figure 1.7   Figure 1.8   Figure 1.9

Figures 1.10–1.13 illustrate different stages of learning to roll from back to tummy.

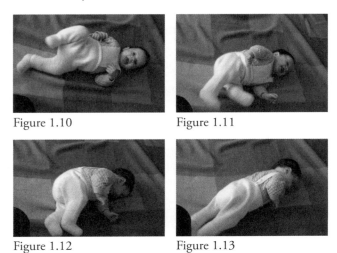

Figure 1.10   Figure 1.11

Figure 1.12   Figure 1.13

Lying on the tummy (when awake*) presents a different set of challenges from lying on the back, partly because the head must either be turned to one side in order to breathe (figure 1.14) and also because the baby needs to learn to lift her head before she can increase her scope of vision (figure 1.15).

Figure 1.14 shows a characteristic posture of the newborn; arms and legs flexed; head turned to one side.

Figure 1.15 shows a baby at about 6 weeks. She is able to lift her head with the back of her head in line with her body. The palmar grasp reflex is still evident in her hands.

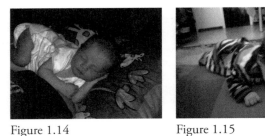

Figure 1.14   Figure 1.15

---

* Advice to parents is that babies should be laid to sleep on their back as this has been found to reduce the incidence of Sudden Infant Death Syndrome (SIDS). This advice has meant that many parents have also stopped placing their baby on the tummy **when awake.** From 3–4 weeks of age, tummy time when awake is important for developing a number of skills.

Learning head control is a lengthy process, and usually begins with a small upward and backward movement of the head off the ground (Figure 1.15). Slowly, as neck muscles strengthen, the hands become more involved in supporting the upper trunk, followed by use of the forearms (Figure 1.22), then the whole arm (Figure 1.23) until she has sufficient upper body control to lift the upper part of her body completely off the ground with legs and feet in the air (the Landau reflex, Figure 1.24).

Figures 1.16–1.22 show increase in head control. In Figure 1.16 for example, the head can now be held above the level of the body and the forearms are involved in supporting the upper body. Palmar (gripping) reflex is still evident in the hands.

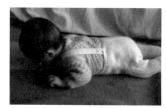

Figure 1.16

In Figures 1.17–1.18 the head can now be held above the level of the body; neck and upper trunk strength developing; Figures 1.19–1.22 show increased use of the forearms and eventually the whole arms in supporting the upper body. Palmar (gripping) reflex is still evident in the hands in the early stages, but recedes as head and upper trunk control increase.

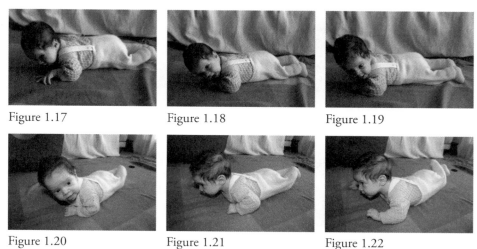

Figure 1.17   Figure 1.18   Figure 1.19

Figure 1.20   Figure 1.21   Figure 1.22

Figure 1.23 illustrates increased head control and use of the forearms for support. Fingers are still partly curled. Lower legs are involved in kicking and punching movements.

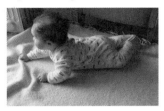

Figure 1.23

Figure 1.23 also shows the emergence of an amphibian reflex in the left leg. This ability to flex one leg or one quadrant of the body independently of other parts of the body is a precursor to being able to crawl on the tummy like a commando, and supports many other coordinated actions in later life.

Figure 1.24. shows the Landau reflex, the ability to elevate head and torso without arm support. The lower legs are also slightly elevated.

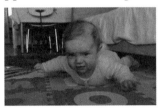

Figure 1.24

Figure 1.25 shows a baby getting ready to roll from tummy to back.

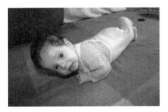

Figure 1.25

In Figure 1.26 she is getting ready to 'commando' crawl.

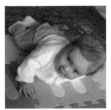

Figure 1.26

Figures 1.27–1.29 show full arm extension used for upper body support. Figure 1.30 shows increasing upper and lower body strength; one arm only is needed for full support, the other is free for reaching and grasping; fingers open. She is able to push with her feet and lower legs, preparing to get up on to hands and knees.

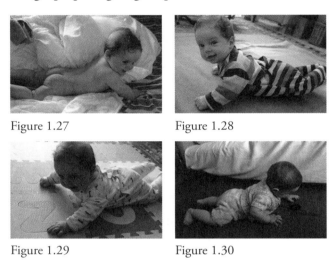

Figure 1.27   Figure 1.28

Figure 1.29   Figure 1.30

In Figure 1.31 she is getting ready to crawl on hands and knees. Symmetrical tonic neck reflex is still evident.

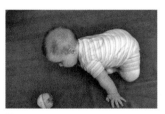

Figure 1.31

In Figures 1.32 and 1.33, infant rocking on hands and knees helps to integrate control of upper and lower body needed for crawling on the hands and knees.

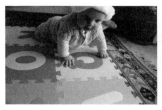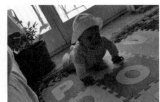

Figure 1.32   Figure 1.33

Figures 1.34–1.36 show the baby learning to sit independently.

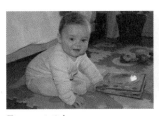
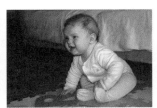
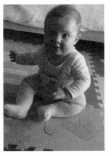

Figure 1.34
Two-armed prop

Figure 1.35
One-arm prop

Figure 1.36
Unsupported sitting

Figures 1.37–1.40 show the beginnings of crawling.

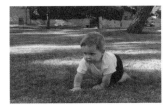
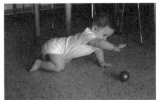

Figure 1.37
Space explorer

Figure 1.38
Moving and reaching

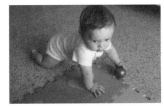
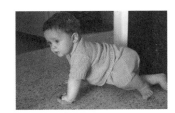

Figure 1.39
Moving and grasping

Figure 1.40
Bear walking

Figures 1.41–1.43 show her getting ready to stand.

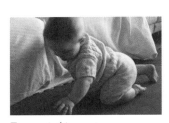
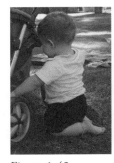
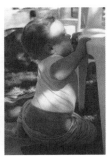

Figure 1.41

Figure 1.42

Figure 1.43

Figures 1.44–1.46 demonstrate the 'Terranaut'.

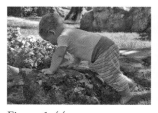
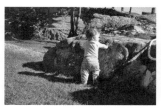
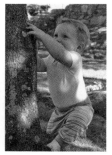

Figure 1.44   Figure 1.45   Figure 1.46

Free movement

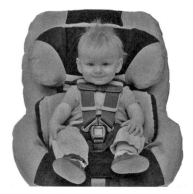

While baby seats are essential for child safety in the car, the opportunity and range of movements a baby is able to experience from the confines of a baby seat are very different from the repertoire available to practise on the floor. There is also a difference between being placed into a sitting position by an adult, and learning how to sit up by yourself. Learning *how* to do some-

Figure 1.47

thing is as important as learning the next postural or motor skill. It also involves the development of sufficient muscle tone and cooperation between different motor centres in planning and carrying out a sequence of movements.

Similarly, baby bouncing cradles may be a godsend to parents for

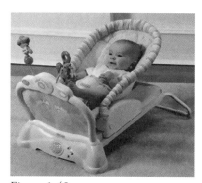

short periods of the day when baby is awake and can be left to play in relative safety, but once again the range of movements available to the baby is restricted, particularly movements involving extension of the head, development of upper body control, and truncal rotation (Figure 1.48).

Figure 1.48

Truncal movements are necessary for twisting, turning and rolling, and facilitating efficient cooperative use of the upper and lower sections of the body (Figure 1.49).

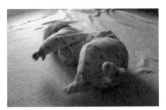

Figure 1.49

Later on, truncal mobility will support fluency of gross motor movements such as running, chasing and kicking a ball, jumping, leaping over an object etc (Figure 1.50).

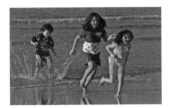

Figure 1.50

The impact of baby equipment is not confined to restricting movement experience. In 2008 a report was published based on an observational study of more than 2,722 parent–infant pairs across the country, which suggested that even the type of buggy used can affect a baby's development. Placed in the context of 21st-century babies potentially experiencing greater physical and social isolation than babies in the past, the study suggested that old-fashioned buggies, which allow babies to lie down and look up at their parent, give babies the best start in life, allowing the baby to see the parent and watch the parent's reactions; and for parent and child to carry on a dialogue when out together. The study found that parents using face-to-face buggies were more than twice as likely to be talking to their child.[11]

A separate, small-scale study observed the behaviour of twenty babies and their parents as they were wheeled in push-chairs across a one-mile stretch of Dundee. Half of the journey was spent in a parent-facing buggy and the other half in an away-facing buggy. The baby's average heart rate fell slightly when in a parent-facing position, and babies were more likely to fall asleep in this position, suggesting that they may be more stressed when in an away-facing position, or more aroused by increased exposure to multiple stimuli without being able to see the parent figure.

Zeedyk emphasized that numbers in the second study were small; but taking this into account,

> If babies are spending significant amounts of time in a baby buggy that undermines their ability to communicate with their parent, at an age when the brain is developing more than it ever will again, then this has to impact negatively on their development. Our experimental study showed that, simply by turning the buggy around, parents' rate of talking to their baby doubled.[12]

Principles of movement development

The majority of children will reach certain milestones such as head control, sitting, walking and talking at predictable times in terms of chronological age. These milestones provide markers of stages of development and are known as developmental *norms,* although *norm* should not be confused with *normal.* This is because every child is an individual and will vary in the rate at which she develops different skills. Cultural differences may also affect this. However, general patterns of expected development can be helpful in looking at a child's development as a whole.

In terms of movement, they are categorized as:

1 Gross motor skills.
2 Fine motor skills.

1 Gross motor skills refer to whole body movements involving posture and larger movements, and follow a predictable sequence:
   - Learning to support the head
   - Learning to support the upper body
   - Rolling
   - Sitting
   - Crawling

- Pulling to stand
- Walking
- Running
- Climbing stairs
- Hopping
- Kicking a ball
- Skipping
- Riding a tricycle and then bicycle
- Swimming*
- Climbing

There is also a general sequence in the development of certain movement patterns beginning with homologous movements – simultaneous, identical flexion or extension of the upper and lower portions of the body with both sides doing the same thing. You might see this when your baby makes her first attempts to crawl on her tummy, trying to pull with both arms and push with both legs. She will be able to move forward using the method, but it takes a lot of effort to make very little progress. She may then try to pull with one arm and push with the leg on the same side. This is described as a homolateral – or one sided movement – and is a little more efficient than homologous crawling but is still not the best way of moving around on the tummy. The most advanced phase is described as cross pattern: when your baby pulls with one arm and pushes with the toes of the opposite leg, like a commando crawling through the grass. Earlier patterns of movement may be seen again each time your baby learns a new style or level of locomotion such as creeping on hands and knees, walking, climbing or later dancing (the dancing partner with two left feet!) Not every child passes through every one of these phases, nor does every child crawl on her tummy or creep on hands and knees.

---

* Babies are also able to swim at birth, but they quickly lose this instinct unless encouraged to use it a few months later. One reason that a baby is able to swim at birth and is adapted to immersion in water is the presence of a mammalian diving reflex that makes them automatically hold their breath whilst submerged. The ideal age to start to re-train your baby to swim is 3–12 months. The minimum age and body weight considered safe is 10 weeks and 10 pounds. The oldest that we can take babies into the water in this way is 18 months

You should not be overly concerned if your baby chooses not to crawl or creep in the first year, provided that you have given her every opportunity to experiment in terms of space and free play. If necessary, these particular modes of locomotion can be introduced into games such as crawling through a tunnel when the child is a little older.

2   Fine motor skills describe movement abilities involving small muscles and precise movement, particularly small movements of the hands, wrists, fingers, feet, toes, lips, and tongue. Fine motor skills are necessary not only for reaching, grasping and manipulation but also for clear articulation. Gross and fine motor skills usually develop together since many activities depend on a combination of gross and fine motor coordination.

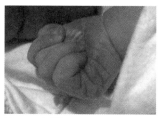

Figure 1.51
Palmar grasp reflex

Development of manipulation provides an example of how fine motor skills are refined in the first years of life, beginning with random opening and closing of the whole hand (the palmar reflex). The palmar reflex describes your baby's reaction if you place a finger inside the palm of his hand and she grasps hold of your finger and will not let go for several seconds. This reflex remains active for several months after birth, affecting the dexterity of hand and finger movements, because the reflex causes *all* of the fingers to close together with the thumb underneath when the palm of the hand is touched. As the nervous system develops, the early reflexes of the newborn are gradually modified and transformed into more mature patterns of response, enabling your baby to develop an increasing repertoire of voluntary movements.*

---

*   There are two main groups of reflexes in the first years of life. The first are called **primitive** reflexes. These are reflexes which developed during life in the womb, and which are modified and transformed in the first 6 months of life as both the nervous and postural systems mature.

The second group of reflexes are called **postural** reflexes. These are reflexes which develop after birth, taking up to three and a half years to mature. They support balance, posture and coordination for the remainder of life.

Indications of the palmar reflex receding include when your baby can open her hands out to support the weight of her upper body when lying on her tummy, and when she starts to drop objects such as toys or food. This is a sign that she is able to 'let go' of an object at will. It is a precursor to being able to use each finger independently and to hold an object between the thumb and forefinger (pincer grip). Grasping movements will develop from attempting to grasp an object using the whole hand, holding and exploring objects, separating thumb from finger movements to a primitive 'pincer' grasp using thumb and forefinger, exploration with the index finger and eventually the ability to use the thumb and forefinger independently from the other fingers.

Reflexes

Normal growth and development involve many phases of change. Babies are born with basic reflexes and life-preserving instincts. These are automatic and carried out at a low level of brain function, as connections to and from higher-level brain structures must be developed through the dual processes of maturation and experience. From basic reflex reactions, a baby begins to develop muscle tone and increased postural control. We have already seen how control of the head position is essential for the smooth execution of all other coordination from grasping to reaching, sitting, standing and control of upright balance. Head control even influences the eventual control of eye movements needed for reading, writing and driving a car!

The transition from early infant (primitive) reflexes to more mature postural reflexes takes up to $3^{1}/_{2}$ years of age, and does not necessarily proceed in a rigid sequence. Rather, every new ability incorporates a previous one, but has a new and higher level of organization. As a baby learns a new postural skill in relation to gravity, she must then practise it many times and calibrate a new position in space with other sensory systems: from passively lying on back or tummy, to sitting, four-point kneeling (crawling position), standing and walking. Once the upright position is achieved, the whole process of learning to move on two legs starts from the beginning again, based on earlier movement patterns. You may therefore witness your baby learn a new skill such as rolling, sitting or crawling, and then appear to get 'stuck' there for a few weeks, content to practise old patterns in new ways. This is why every stage of your child's development matters, and you should not be tempted to hurry her through one stage to 'catch up' with another child of a similar age. Each stage is important in securing and integrating previously learned skills, and each child progresses at her own rate.

A child goes through many phases of change in the first three years of life, when development and maturation of the central nervous system proceed at a faster rate than they will at any other time in life. A child learns more in the first six years of life through interaction and play than she will in a lifetime of formal study. A quotation attributed to the Jesuit Francis Xavier states: 'Give me a child until he is seven and I will give you the man', highlighting the decisive influence of the first six years of life. A.A. Milne put it slightly differently when Christopher Robin said, 'Now I am six I'm as clever as clever. I think I'll stay six now forever and ever.'[13]

Outdoor play

As your baby gets older, time spent in outdoor play is just as important as indoor play. The sounds, smells, sights, textures and temperature are completely different when playing outdoors, as is the amount of space and materials available for exploration and discovery. The type of exercise outdoor play encourages is generally more robust, involving more extensive use of balance and gross motor activities than indoor play.

Try to find or create an area outdoors where it is safe for your child to play. For safety reasons, the younger the child, the more restricted the area is likely to be. In the first 6 months of life this may just be a rug placed on the grass in the summer months within close sight and sound of an adult; once your baby becomes mobile, a contained area such as a playpen or small, enclosed yard is ideal.

As your toddler becomes more adventurous, outdoor play should be within easy physical reach of an adult but still provide enough scope for exploration and adventure within the child's developmental capabilities. If you do not have a garden, or only a small outdoor play area, try to take your child for a walk or to the park at least three days a week. If your child cannot walk that far, use a toy with wheels which she can propel along the pavement using her feet.

As your child gets older, rough outdoor play areas are just as good as formal play equipment since they provide a variety of textures, surfaces and gradients to explore. Climbing up a muddy bank and then sliding or rolling down is just as much fun and provides much more tactile stimulation than going down a slide – although it may also create more washing! Trees and bushes make ideal settings for games of hide-and-seek, climbing, sliding and jumping. Just a pile of leaves and sticks can provide all the materials for building a den.

I had three children in less than four years. When they were collectively aged between two and six, I remember taking them to play on some common grazing land. The land had lots of grassy hollows, mounds and dips, with some old iron railings originally used for sheep pens which had been discarded in one of the hollows. They spent an entire day with four small sections of iron railing and straw, building a house. They still talk about this day twenty years later. For them the 'house' with all its holes in the roof was real, and their imaginations ran free for many happy hours. Further up the hill there were several copses of trees. The upper branches of one tree had entwined to form the shape of an upside-down umbrella. If you could manage to climb up the short trunk, there was a gap you could slide through, and the knotted branches formed a natural tree house. I had played in the same tree when I was a child – learning to climb, slide through the space, and slither down again was like a rite of passage, showing I was old enough to join the secret world of older children inside the tree house to which adults were only admitted by invitation.

Outdoor play encourages children to gain mastery and confidence in the use of their bodies. While safety should always be the first consideration, unless children learn to take small risks, to make minor mistakes and learn how to avoid them or correct them for themselves, they cannot gain full confidence in the use of the body. Over-protectiveness, which restricts children's physical experience, can stunt not only their physical but also emotional development. It can create a climate of fear about trying new situations, assessing risks and developing self-sufficiency.

Outdoor play provides opportunity to run and to shout; to play with water, sand and mud without the mess being a problem; to fill containers and start to learn through physical experience about volume and quantity; to run, ride and make things on an uneven surface; and to understand how different types of surface behave in different ways. A larger space in which to play helps children learn about distance, space, speed and time (the sense of time develops partly from discovering how long it takes to get from point to point), and enables them to use long-distance vision to the full, something which is not developed watching television or playing a computer game.

The outdoors provides a backdrop for dramatic play emerging from the child's own imagination. This is the world in which the child can be heroic and involve other children as the dramatis persona in her private domain. When I was growing up, there were three fir trees of varying size in our garden, each one with a branch just high enough to climb on to safely. My middle sister was mad about horses and led the three of us in hair-raising adventures, using the branches as imaginary horses which we rode to save maidens in distress, deliver messages to the general, and round up cattle on the ranch. All of this was possible without ever leaving the safety of the garden.

More formal play settings where equipment such as slides, swings, climbing apparatus and riding toys are provided also afford opportunity to develop balance, muscle tone and coordination. Vigorous exercise of any kind improves respiration and increases circulation. Activity is necessary to help nutrients work their way efficiently through the body so that we derive optimum uptake and energy from the food we eat. Children are no different from adults in this respect.

Outdoor play is also important in northern temperate zones to provide exposure to sunlight throughout the year. The United Kingdom is in a latitude where the amount of sunlight received during the winter months is only sufficient in the south of the country (south of Birmingham) for providing the amount of vitamin D needed for healthy growth, bone development and immune functioning. Sunlight is the main source of vitamin D. While it can also be obtained from dietary sources such as fish and fortified milk, time spent playing in full daylight and fresh air helps to maintain vitamin D levels, particularly in the winter months, enabling the body to absorb the calcium that is essential for healthy bone development.

Outdoor play can be adjusted to the space available. Large spaces make free play easier, but even a relatively small area can be used and adults can help children find ways of using the space for maximum activity. Here are just a few examples:

- Running to a target and back again
- Cross the space making swimming movements with the arms
- Marching
- Hopping
- Skipping
- Walking and running on tip-toes
- Running and jumping on the spot
- Stretching up and down and from side to side
- Place an object such as a hoop on the ground. Tell the children to run around the outside, in one direction and then in the other; tell them to jump inside the hoop and then out of it; tell them to pretend the hoop is the opening to a deep hole and climb into it; then climb out.

With a little imagination and minimum equipment the possibilities are endless! Many children will go on to devise their own games without the need for adult-led activities.

Rough and tumble play

A climate of fear surrounding issues of child abuse and child safety has meant that in recent years children placed in nursery care tend to receive less experience of touch than in previous generations, both in the form of adult touch and the touch and feedback derived from rough and tumble play. Studies with animals have found that rough and tumble play is an essential ingredient of healthy development and socialization in animal groups. Animal pups deprived of physical interaction show withdrawn, antisocial and aggressive behaviour. On the one hand, insufficient sensory experience can result in sensation-seeking or avoidance behaviour; and on the other, not allowing children to take reasonable risks and experience the consequences in childhood can make them more prone to indulging in high-risk behaviour or, conversely, being overly fearful of taking risks or trying new situations later on. Rough and tumble play in the early years provides a wealth of tactile experience as well as developing physical fitness, sensory awareness, regulation of strength and self-control, and inviting flexible and creative behaviour.[14]

Early years education in Finland

The reason for including a short section on pre-school provision in Finland at this point is because it provides a 'gold standard' in terms of its emphasis on parental involvement, flexibility in childcare options, physical interaction, outdoor play and learning through (guided) experience until formal schooling begins at around seven years of age.

Parents have the option of three types of childcare until the child begins compulsory schooling:

1   Caring for the child at home on care leave and receiving child home-care allowance.
2   Having the child cared for in private daycare with private child-care allowance.
3   Having the child cared for in municipal day-centres.

In the year before starting compulsory schooling, when the child is six, the child can enter pre-school education. This is provided by the local authority for 700 hours during the academic year, but is still optional. The ratio of adults to children is 1.7 for 3–6 year olds and 1.4 for children under the age of three in full daycare. In all Finnish pre-school care, growing and learning are understood to constitute a lifelong process. The principle aims of the curriculum as described in a leaflet produced by the Ministry of Social Affairs and Health in Helsinki are:

> To promote the child's overall well-being so as to ensure the best possible conditions for growth, learning and development. Hence the child is able to enjoy the company of others, experiencing joy and freedom of action in an unhurried, safe atmosphere.

The child is an active learner whose learning is guided by curiosity, the will to explore and joy of realization. The core of learning is the interaction between children, adults and the environment. To this end, the environment should be versatile. Nature and the immediate neighbourhood are important elements of the environment, and the environment enables the use of all senses and the whole body for play, movement, expression, experimentation and insights.

Playing, movement, exploration and self-expression through different forms of art are ways of acting and thinking peculiar to children. Parents have the primary right to and responsibility for their child's education. They also know their child best. Therefore, the educators have a key role in sharing the day-to-day education and care of the young child with the parents.[15]

A typical day for the pre-school child in Finland takes physical and developmental needs into account. Some children may arrive as early as 7 a.m., but the formal day begins at 8 a.m.:

8–8.30	Breakfast time.
8.30	Morning meeting of children. As a group, children talk about what has happened in the calendar and what they are going to do today; read a story or sing together.
9–10	Work activities.
10–11	Outdoor play.
11	Circle time – reading a book or singing together
11.30–12	Lunch. Some children may go home after lunch.
12–12.30	General story time.
1–2	Rest or sleep time. A special rest area is provided.
2	Snack.
2.30–3.30	Indoor play to finish things off as concentration tends to drop off at this time of day.
3.30–5	Outdoor play (unless the weather is very bad).

Children are equipped with suitable clothing for outdoor play in all weathers, and plenty of outdoor space and toys are provided. The only time children will not go out to play is if the temperature falls below –15 degrees centigrade! There is also a rest area provided where children can snuggle down on a small bed with a blanket for the set 'rest period' in the early afternoon.

This pre-school model takes the developmental needs of the pre-school child into account, recognizing the prime role taken by parents, allowing flexibility and choice in childcare arrangements, encouraging physical play and exploration, and only insisting on formal instruction in reading and writing from age seven. While some children seem eager and able to start reading from as young as four, others take a good deal longer. This is because individual rate of maturation can vary. Boys for example are generally slightly later than girls in developing fine motor skills. This can include speech and language as well as the more obvious fine motor skills needed to hold and control a pencil. They also tend to need more opportunity for gross motor activities in the day, which can make it harder for them to sit still and concentrate for long periods of time. Reading requires not only the ability to hear and distinguish the minute differences between similar sounds such as *b* and *d, m* and *n, th* and *f, sh* and *ch* etc. but also, sufficient control of eye movements to follow along a line of print without the eyes jumping further along the line, to the line above or the line below. This can easily take up to age seven to develop, and is partly dependent on the functioning of head-righting reflexes needed to provide a stable platform upon which centres involved in the control of eye movements rely for stable support.

A series of studies carried out in schools in England and Northern Ireland between 2001 and 2005 found that there was a link between immature physical skills and lower educational achievement in a group of five- to six-year-old children.[16] In other words, physical development supports higher 'thinking' skills and the ability to express knowledge in ways required in the classroom. Remember that every stage of development is incorporated into a higher stage, but with increased organization and efficiency. If the physical foundations have been securely laid in the early years, children are better able to reveal their potential when formal education begins.

In a nutshell

Movement experience in the early years matters because

- Movement is the primary medium through which sensory integration takes place.

- Movement experience helps a child to develop an internal body map.
- Movement helps a child to know her place and position in space. This forms the basis or reference point from which other spatial judgements are made.
- In the first years of life, emotional regulation is felt and expressed in physical ways and is derived from touch, feeding, movement experience, social engagement and rough and tumble play.
- Confidence in using the body develops non-verbal aspects of language and the ability to understand the non-verbal language of others.
- Outdoor play is important for developing balance, coordination and imagination. It also has a number of health benefits.
- Rough and tumble play invites children to act and play in creative ways; it helps to develop self-regulation, self-control and is an essential part of healthy development in all young mammals.
- Sensations derived from exercising the balance mechanism help to train centres in the brain involved in the control of eye movements, necessary for reading, writing, copying and physical education later on.
- Movement has the capacity to soothe or arouse and is usually a joyful experience for young children. When there is joy, children learn.[17]

Notes

1   E.J. Kiphard: 'Psychiatrist clown relieves children's fears.' Article received via personal communication. 1980.
2   A.N. Meltzoff, M.K. Moore: 'Imitation of facial and manual gestures by human neonates.' *Science* 198: 75–8 1977.
3   A.N. Meltzoff, M.K. Moore: 'Newborn infants imitate adults' facial gestures.' *Child Development* 54: 702–9 1983.
4   R.H. Barsch: *Achieving Perceptual-Motor Efficiency. A Space Oriented Approach to Learning. Volume 1 of a perceptual-motor curriculum.* Special Child Publications, Seattle WA 1968.
5   S. Mines: 'I Can Feel My Baby Move! Prenatal Developmental Movement and Parental Response.' http://www.selfgrowth.com/articles/Mines1.html
6   http://www.babyhut.co.uk/
7   M.F. Small: *Our Babies Ourselves. How Biology and Culture Shape the Way we Parent.* Anchor Books, New York 1999.

8 A. Schore: *Affect Regulation and the Origin of the Self.* Laurence Erlbaum, Hove 1994.

9 E. Haeckel: *Riddle of the Universe at the Close of the Nineteenth Century.* 1899.

10 S.A. Goddard Blythe: *What Babies and Children Really Need.* Hawthorn Press, Stroud 2008.

11 S. Zeedyk: 'Talk to your baby.' Baby buggies may undermine child development. National Literacy Trust, 21.11.2008.

12 S. Zeedyk. Cited in: Curtis, P: 'Type of buggy can affect baby development, study finds.' *The Guardian* 21.11.2008.

13 A.A. Milne: *Now We Are Six.* Methuen and Company, London 1927.

14 J. Panksepp: *Affective Neuroscience: The Foundations of Human and Animal Emotions.* Oxford University Press, New York 1998.

15 'Early childhood education and care in Finland'. Brochures of the Ministry of Social Affairs and Health 2004: 14. Helsinki, Finland.

16 S.A. Goddard Blythe: 'Releasing educational potential through movement. A summary of individual studies carried out using the INPP test battery and developmental exercise programme for use in schools with children with special needs.' *Child Care in Practice.* 11/4: 415–32. 2005.

17 E.J. Kiphard: 'Intervention programmes using the German psycho-motor approach with exceptional children.' Paper presented at The 12th European Conference of Neuro-Developmental Delay in Children with Specific Learning Difficulties. Chester, March 2000.

CHAPTER 2

Music and Language

Mime and music

The development of language in the early years also involves the practice of two crucial elements – gesture and music – that have been intrinsic to human life from its most ancient beginnings. Long before a child learns to speak he communicates using sounds and gestures. Cooing and babbling are essentially musical in nature, and the hand movements and gestures made by infants engaged in both listening and vocalizing have been compared to the highly trained hand movements of an orchestral conductor.[1] Nearly 150 years ago, Charles Darwin wrote: 'I have been led to infer that the progenitors of man probably uttered musical tones before they had acquired the powers of articulate speech.'[2]

What we think of as music in the modern world has its origins in two types of sound: the first is rhythm, which in early times was expressed through movement and actions – body-based communication – such as the beating of drums, ritual and dance movements and the stamping of feet. Rhythm is articulated through pathways which involve touch, balance, proprioception and action. The second type is tone – sounds made with the vocal organs, and often associated with nature and human activities such as hunting calls, animal cries and bird-calls. These two, simple types of utterance are controlled by primitive parts of the brain, which are more active in infancy than the ones which later govern speech. In other words, rhythmical and musical centres of the brain are more 'ready for use' in the early years than higher centres, whose many connections need to be formed over time to support speech and written language. In this respect, in the early years music is the pre-verbal expression of language and prepares the ear, voice and brain for speech.

Babies are born with an innate desire to communicate. Communication begins before birth when the unborn child is able to feel his mother's emotions in a number of different ways: for example through chemical changes that take place in her body in response to her environment and mood, alterations in the nature and speed of her physiological functions such as heart-rate and breathing, changes in the speed and force of her bodily movements, and the over-riding accompaniment provided by the melody, timbre and rhythms of her voice. The unborn child is able to detect elements of the mother's speech through a combination of vibration and sound. Vibration is particularly important because the pre-birth environment is aqueous, and thus the sounds of the outside world are filtered through a combination of amniotic fluid and the protective barrier of the mother's body. After birth, sounds are conducted to the hearing apparatus in the inner ear through the dual media of air and bone, whereas before birth the foetus can only hear sounds relayed through bone conduction. The range of sounds transmitted through bone conduction is limited to lower frequencies.

From the 24th week of pregnancy babies can 'hear' – but only a restricted range of lower- to medium-frequency sounds, which roughly correspond to the range of the human voice and the majority of musical instruments used in classical music. All sounds heard inside the womb are reduced in volume by about thirty per cent, the loudest sound being that of the mother's heartbeat. Sounds from the outside world are about 35 decibels quieter than sounds generated from the internal environment. *The only exception is the sound of the mother's voice,* which is particularly powerful because it resonates internally and externally, her body acting as the sounding board. A woman's body is designed to be the perfect resonator of sound before birth for this range of low to middle frequencies. The sound of her voice, in the tones, melodies and rhythms of her speech, provides a kind of acoustic massage to the unborn child. According to French-Canadian director of The Listening Centre in Toronto, P. Madaule, there is a good reason why a cello is shaped like the human body:

'The shape and contours that form the body of the instrument make the perfect sound resonator.'[3]

Figures 2.1 and 2.2 below illustrate the similarity between the shape of a woman's body and the shape of stringed instruments in which the 'body' of the instrument acts as the sound resonator.

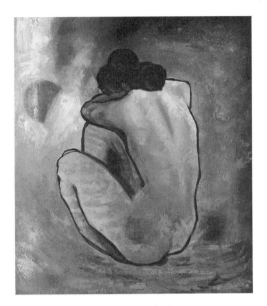

Figure 2.1 'Blue Nude' by Picasso

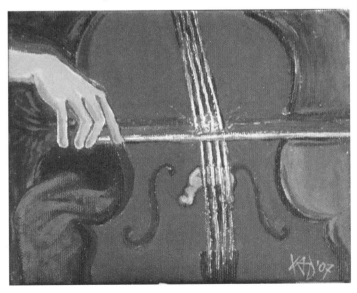

Figure 2.2

Lazarev's theory of pre-natal development

Michael Lazarev, a Russian physician and musician, has developed a theory of pre-natal development and a method of musical education designed to be used by parents and child from the third trimester of pregnancy up to seven years of age. 'Every mother,' he says, 'should be a professional mother – you are the real guardian angel of your child'.[4] In this sense, every mother is a child's first teacher. Specialist educators, therapists and physicians are only there to *support* parents in specific aspects of their child's upbringing, not replace them.

The prenatal child is provided with a vast supply of neurons, only a fraction of which will be used during his lifetime. This over-production of prenatal brain neurons is an evolutionary mechanism thought to prepare human beings, originally designed to live in a very different environment from the one we live in today, to experience and adapt to the sensory demands of a world which changes with each generation and throughout a person's lifespan. Lazarev believes one way of preparing the unborn child for his new world is by introducing him to the world of sound before birth, using the universal language of music as the medium and the mother's voice as the instrument.

In his earlier professional life Lazarev worked as a doctor in a medical centre specializing in the treatment of children with bronchial asthma and other respiratory diseases. He developed a programme of remedial gymnastics for children with asthma, and noticed that both asthma and diseases associated with periods of very cold temperature improved when patients took part in musical activities including singing. He concluded that musical participation must strengthen the immune system, and recognized that music alters our emotional state through its relationship with respiratory function.

Speech and singing have a powerful effect not only on the immune system but also on other physiological processes including cardio-respiratory function, digestion, hormonal secretion, motion, emotion and intelligence. Both before and after birth, a mother's voice provides a connection between respiration, sound and movement – an acoustic link between pre-birth life and the brave new world after birth:

> Mama's voice is the main instrument in his pre-natal education. This is a tuning fork to attune the strings of the soul to vibrations

of the outside world, to get into a universe of human culture. These vibrations are the first to form the deepest structures of his personality.[5]

Mother, he says, 'is the sculptor who shapes her baby with her voice', both before and after birth. Music is the natural medium for this creative and connective process, because it is composed of elements which are common to all languages, all forms of communication, and can be understood at a physical and emotional level by the very young child.

Music and speech share many elements in common: the separation of sounds into individual sounds or sound streams which convey emotional meaning; the prosody, or rhythmic structure of language including stress and intonation; pitch, beat or pulse, which provide an underlying sense of structure in time and space; rhythm, which describes the measure of expressive movements in time; and the different tensions that can be created by changing or combining rhythms. The rhythm of a melody is often based on the inflections of language, the physical rhythms of dance, or simply periodic pulsation. Melody is typically divided into *phrases* within a larger overarching structure, which roughly correspond to breathing spaces in speech and punctuation in written language.

Melody and key have a powerful influence on mood and atmosphere, while harmony provides colour, depth and texture. The combined effect of melody, harmony and rhythm create tension, anticipation, emotional longing, and a deep sense of resolution, evoking the whole range of human emotions. The music of language is conveyed through the melodic, rhythmic and expressive qualities that underlie interaction and meaning in human communication. While the meaning of words can be interpreted in many different ways *depending on the manner* in which they are delivered, it is these non-verbal aspects of *delivery* which are essentially musical in nature, and which form the vital ingredients of effective communication. Children are ready to listen, learn and perform the music of language long before they are ready to speak.

Babies and infants (infant originally means 'one without speech') naturally have a special language that is more akin to music and mime than to speech, but they also need a receptive and responsive audience to develop this special language. The importance of audience participation in the development of communication was illustrated by research carried out at the University of Edinburgh,[6] which examined mother–infant interactions in the first weeks of life. The researchers discovered that when a mother was attuned and responsive to her baby, a dialogue takes place in which the mother utters short phrases to her baby in a sing-song voice. If she waits for a few seconds, the baby will sing an answering phrase in return. When the dialogue was analysed using a sound-frequency analyser, the conversation showed all the features of a musical composition – melody, structured timing, phrasing and cadence – with one partner repeating and answering the musical phrase of the other. If the adult 'interrupted' the baby before he had time to reply, the baby gave up and the 'conversation' came to an end. Even at this very young age, babies seem to understand the importance of listening and the etiquette of conversation. Adults are not always so polite! It seems that the human infant really does learn to dance before he can walk, and to sing long before he can talk.

The special language used by adults with young babies is called 'motherese'. One of the main characteristics of motherese is that it is slower than normal speech. Utterances are shorter and more regularly spaced, with short intervals. Mother and infant communicate using a shared tempo, and the essential features of communication between the two are based on intonation contours (melody) and on reciprocal taking of turns. This is very similar to what happens in singing. Even in birds, the development of song involves the vocal duplication of an auditory model, and birds like humans have a developmental lag between first hearing sounds and later being able to reproduce them and becoming vocally competent performers. This has led to the sub-song (listening and practice phase) of avian development being compared to the babbling phase of human development.[6]

Dance and dialogue

Building on these early, innate abilities is partly dependent on receiving sufficient and appropriate environmental experience in the form of social engagement – first with the primary source of love, and later with siblings, adults and peers. The first months of life are when lullabies, nursery rhymes, songs and action games naturally provide a means of welcoming every infant into the accents, traditions and heritage of his culture. Just as every language uses a range of sounds unique to that language, so the lullabies, songs and rhymes of every culture carry within them the 'signature' melodies and inflections of the mother tongue, preparing the ear, the voice and the brain for speech.

The technological revolution of the past thirty years, and the lifestyle changes it has brought with it, are already having a profound impact on the quality and quantity of direct, one-to-one communication with children. Entertainment provided by electronic media may be useful for short periods of time to soothe, occupy or entertain a fretful child, but it cannot provide the same rich experiences derived from direct, interactive communication with another person.

Social interaction with another involves the ability to 'read', replicate and reproduce all the nuances and subtleties gleaned from their body language and spontaneous responses. Stimulation derived from a remote or virtual source provides stimulation, but does not listen to what the child has to say, neither does it adapt to the child's moment-to-moment needs. It is essentially an egotistical form of communication which follows its own course without consideration for the listener or the viewer. This medium of stimulation occurs in a pre-programmed, virtual world with pre-set responses created by a particular type of mind – the mind of a computer software designer. In other words it offers monologue, not dialogue.

Reciprocal communication is an essential feature of empathy – to feel as another – and recent research has confirmed a long-held observation that people who share a close relationship seem to be 'on the same wavelength'. Dr Trisha Stratford of the University of Technology in Sydney studied the brains and heartbeats of thirty volunteers during counselling sessions. She identified a crucial moment when the brains and heart rates of the counsellor and patient started to function in synchrony and they became attuned to one another's thoughts.[7] Similar patterns have been found in couples who start to think like each other, enabling them to know what their partner is thinking or about to say. The more closely attuned a parent is to their child, the more likely they are to be able to respond in a positive way to his behaviour, whether good or bad. This is similar to the example mentioned in Chapter 1 of the non-verbal communication which exists between mother and child in many indigenous cultures, where carrying connects the child physically to the mother during the first months of life. Music and the sharing of live music also support a sense of feeling and communicating as one.

How does music teach language?

'We live, think, imagine and remember in movement.'[8] Even thought is an internalized form of action,[9] and music embodies movement in sound. Making music also entails movement, the sounds of music being inseparable from carrying out and controlling actions. In this way musical expression is the natural sequel and accompaniment to the development of movement control in infancy. The sharing of music with others trains cooperative behaviour through the inference of underlying pulse and anticipation of movement. Like speech, music is communicated through controlled bodily movement, and involves the selection and reproduction of specific sounds and rhythms to convey emotion and meaning.

Music, particularly song, can therefore be used to lay the ground for the next episode of language development. Song is important because it is a special type of speech. Like motherese, it slows down the sounds of speech as we noted, extending the time value of 'open' vowel sounds so that they can be more easily picked up. Streams of sound are separated into short, regularly spaced phrases with pauses between each phrase, making them easier to remember. Words or segments of words are often repeated, helping to build memory of relevant sounds and emphasis or 'stress', which carries an increased time value and is placed on the key syllable in each word that conveys meaning. (Small differences in where the stress or the accent is placed on a word or part of a phrase also constitute major differences between languages. For example in English, the word *coffee* places the stress on the first syllable in the word, whereas in French the stress and accent is placed on the last syllable *café*.)

Singing helps to build a vocabulary of sounds and words long before a child understands precisely what the words mean. Something similar happens to cathedral choristers who learn to vocally reproduce the sounds of complex music and language which is often far in advance of their actual reading age. A former Master of Choristers at Chester Cathedral remarked that 'the reading age of all my boys is at least six months ahead of their chronological age within six months of joining the choir, irrespective of whether they were good or poor readers when they first joined.'[10] His explanation for this was that the process of voicing aloud or 'sounding out' helps to match the vocal sounds formed with the mouth to the visual symbols on the page, helping to develop reading ability without direct instruction.

Use of the child's own voice is also one of the most powerful instruments of learning.[11] Paul Madaule, echoing the words of his mentor Dr. A. Tomatis, has said that the voice can only reproduce what the ear can hear; but he goes on to add that the human ear is continuously enriched and entrained through feedback from the voice to the ear, something he describes as 'the audio-vocal feedback loop'.[12] Children between the ages of three and five often engage in private speech (talking to themselves) when playing alone or when they are absorbed in imaginary play. This normal developmental stage of sub-vocalization is important for being able to think and reason silently later on, as if having a conversation inside the head. Anthony Storr, author of *Music and the Mind*, observed that good readers seem to have developed an 'internal voice' which they hear inside their head when reading silently. Poor readers do not seem to acquire this 'inner voice', relying instead almost entirely on visual scanning of material.[13] Visual scanning, a rapid process, is useful for picking up the gist of text but tends to miss out detail, particularly the finer details of spelling. Reading aloud is a slower process which permits more efficient detection of errors.

Older children and adults often use sub-vocalization and repetition as dual means of committing new facts to memory, as when trying to memorize a new telephone number. The 'inner voice' is also an essential tool in problem solving and regulating one's own behaviour. When I have a dilemma or a problem to resolve I often find myself having 'a conversation inside my head' as one part of my mind reasons and 'tells' the other not to react in a certain way. This is an important part of being able to control impulses and impose reason to inhibit reaction. Psychologists have sometimes described this inner voice as the 'parent within'. Children with poor impulse control, who need to talk excessively, lack not only the capacity for self-restraint but also the ability to hear and pay attention to their 'inner voice'. The inner voice enables us to think with words and reason in silence. These later developmental abilities are rooted in early vocal experience. 'Sounding out' in the early years is a precursor to being able to think with words.

Nursery rhymes and lullabies

The repeated use of rhyming or chiming words, both within and at the end of a line, is a regular feature of nursery rhymes. This helps to develop the ability to discriminate minute differences between similar sounds and understand how minute changes alter meaning.

> _Twin-_ kle, _twin-_ kle, _li-_ ttle _star,_
> _How_ I _won-_ der _what_ you _are._

When we sing lullabies we educate the earliest of the developing senses: the vestibular sense which is acutely sensitive to movement, any change in direction or speed of movement, or to when movement stops and starts; and which is generally soothed or 'lulled' by continuous gentle rocking, swinging or swaying movements. Rocking movements simulate the motion of the mother's walking rhythm, the pre-birth memory of which is familiar and comforting to the infant. The sense of touch is gently stimulated by vibrations produced by her voice, and the sense of hearing through tone, timbre, repetition of similar sounds and the prolongation of certain speech sounds. Lullabies act as a multi-sensory link from pre-natal experience to the new, outside world.

As stated earlier, traditional lullabies and nursery rhymes are important because they contain the specific melodies, stresses and accents peculiar to the language and the culture from which they grew (the music of the language). In this sense lullabies, which contain a universal pattern of movement (rocking, swinging and swaying) help to welcome the child into the language of his culture.

As we also saw, singing extends the time value of the 'open' or vowel sounds in speech. Examination of individuals with dyslexia carried out in the United States showed that in dyslexia the sounds of speech are processed more slowly than normal,[14] meaning that many of the vowel sounds are simply not heard or are perceived in a scrambled form. This is rather like the experience of listening to someone speaking a foreign language of which you have only limited knowledge. It usually sounds as if it is being spoken far too fast. This is because the uneducated ear is slower at processing a stream of unfamiliar sounds and cannot tell where one word ends and the next one begins. The ability to hear vowel sounds does not come naturally to everyone and can feature as a problem in some specific learning difficulties. Complex computerised training programmes have been developed which artificially slow down the sounds of speech, and the child has to carry out repetition exercises, with the speech sounds gradually being speeded up. Singing does a similar thing without the need for the programme, by allocating a longer time value to the vowel sounds.

Singing and chant provide a natural medium for learning to hear and reproduce all the sounds within a word. An example of this dual process can be seen in the words of one of the Christian evening prayers. When this prayer is *intoned* rather than simply said, the space and timing of each word is stretched out, lending additional emotional meaning to powerful words. In this sense, ancient chants are rather like a form of 'motherese' for adults.

De–fend us from the fé–ar of our en–em–ies.

Sound is transitory, passing in a moment, and so must be *remembered.* Music helps speech sounds to remain in the memory for longer as well as providing an access 'key' for retrieval of auditory stimuli. For example, if someone starts to hum the tune I can still remember the words of hymns I learned to sing at nursery school more than fifty years ago. Without the tune I cannot remember any of the words beyond the first line. As a small child I also learned the alphabet to a tune, multiplication tables to rhythmic speech, days of the week, months of the year, vowels and musical notation to rhymes. In other words, music helps both in committing words to memory but also acts as a key to opening the memory store.

Music uses and develops both sides of the brain. Although most of the population have their main language centre in the left side of the brain, in the early years, when language is developing, both sides of the brain are much more involved in language. On the right side of the brain is an area which mirrors many of the properties and connections of speech that take place on the left, but which is given over to singing rather than words alone. Neuro-imaging has shown that music involves more than just centralized hot spots in the brain, occupying large swathes on both sides. 'Nouns and verbs are very different from tones and chords and harmony, but the parts of the brain that process them overlap.'[15]

Other researchers have found that the very brain functions that are enhanced in musicians are often found to be defective in dyslexia and other hindrances to learning, and that musical experience and training enhances skills involved in learning to be listeners, readers and speakers.[16] Dr Nina Kraus of North Western University in Evanston, Illinois has confirmed that, unsurprisingly, musicians can pick out and follow a voice in a crowd better than non-musicians, and that, 'their brains respond distinctly to the specific part of a baby's cry already known to convey the most emotional content to a parent',[17] enabling them to understand more easily the meaning of even primitive forms of communication.

As a parent, even if you do not think you can sing or play a musical instrument, your baby is not a music critic! He will still enjoy and learn from the sounds of your voice. Your voice is a stringed as well as a wind musical instrument and has characteristics which are unique to you. These characteristics comprise *range, rhythm, resonance, register* and the *individual time patterns* that make your voice as individual as your fingerprints.

Good vibrations

The effect of live as opposed to recorded music on living beings has been investigated and illustrated by Professor Yair Schiftan, a former veterinary surgeon who has developed a therapeutic method called Musica Medica. This system provides simultaneous stimulation of sound to the ears and vibrations applied to the skin via two vibrators placed on various parts of the body. In his latest book,[18] Schiftan explains how the combined effect of sound and vibration – which is felt primarily through the tactile sensory channel – means that music is not only heard, but also received as vibration in the same way as during a live concert in a concert hall, or when playing a musical instrument oneself. The effect is like a gentle form of massage with sound acting as the masseur:

> There is a common conviction that music is received only through the aural channel, but music is also felt through skin receptors, which are sensitive to acoustic phenomena at frequencies from 10 to 1000 Hz. The combination of aural stimulation *and* vibrations received through the sense of touch enhances the brain reaction to the stimulus.

He goes on to say that

> ... music is a phenomenon that the human brain decodes particularly well, because music provides an acoustic reflection of emotions, spiritual condition and the performer's movements. These are elements which are communicated directly to the recipient. When transmission is enhanced with the vibratory layer, it increases the brain's activity, involving not only the nervous, but also circulatory, respiratory and muscular systems.

In other words, when a mother or father sings to their child they stimulate far more than just the sense of hearing.

Brain activation derived from musical stimulation also stimulates the production of neurotransmitters – substances which act as the chemical messengers, by means of which the nervous system communicates. 'Dopamine is one example,' writes Schiftan. 'One of the functions of dopamine is as an action motivator, and use of *Musica Medica* also increases secretion of endorphins, which contribute to better wellbeing and pain relief.' In other words, the vibratory effects of live music can affect our neuro-chemistry.

Music is also processed (hearing, understanding and structure) by the same centres in the brain that are responsible for speech and language – the hearing centres, Broca's area and Wernicke's area. Schiftan suggests that this indicates that listening to music can also be a form of speech training and that listening to songs and lyrics can improve pronunciation and enrich vocabulary.

While babies and young children can be soothed to sleep by playing recordings of lullabies and familiar music, the effects of a live performance go much deeper. As far as your baby is concerned, *you* are the musical maestro and *your* voice is his favourite instrument.

The child's own voice a powerful instrument of learning

After your voice, the most powerful teaching instrument is a child's *own* voice. Colin Lane, a former teacher of the deaf, found that even in deaf children clarity of speech and articulation improve when they first listen to the sound of their own voice through a recording device, and then speak along with it. He has been able to improve not only the speech of hearing-impaired children using this method, but also the literacy skills of children with reading, writing and spelling difficulties through the use of a system called ARROW, which utilizes the child's voice.[19] He also found that children pay more attention to the sound of their own voice than to any other – something which will not surprise many parents of highly vocal children!

A music teacher's perspective on the importance of music in the early years

One way to ensure a child has plenty of vocal experience in the early years is through singing. The following section was contributed by Arlette Overman, Voices Foundation Advisory Teacher, Consultant to Hertfordshire Music Service and Director of Red Lion Music. It gives a music teacher's perspective on the importance of singing throughout childhood.

Every child should and can learn to sing, but sadly it may be that those who have not been exposed to singing under the age of seven may never discover their own singing voice. Being able to sing can usually be explained in exactly the same way as being able to talk. If you spend much of your time under the age of three years (including in the womb), listening to 'in tune' singing, the chances are, unless you have a vocal constraint, that you will teach yourself how to produce the notes that you hear and, whilst learning to talk, you will also learn to sing.

Unfortunately, whilst all children of normal ability who have heard a spoken language over a period of three years will start to use it confidently by mimicking what they have heard with an exact copy of dialect, if these same children have not heard good, 'in tune' singing, they will not be able to reproduce it. In many cultures, singing and dancing is part and parcel of growing up. But in the western world this is sadly no longer the case. I recently heard a dreadful rendition of 'Happy birthday to you' in a restaurant by a group of teenagers. Clearly these children had not grown up hearing it correctly (it has to be said that this is a very difficult melody, spanning eight different pitches). I shuddered to think that they would pass on their memory of how the melody goes to their own children and I realized that we have already sadly arrived at a society of 'out of tune' singers who either realize it sounds wrong and therefore shy away from singing completely, or sing with gusto out of tune.

Little children need, in the first place, to hear a wide variety of songs and nursery rhymes from their own culture. This is a perfect way to start listening as, in the case of English, they mimic the rise and falling patterns of a complicated, compound rhythmic language.

I must stress here that the melodies from these well-known rhymes are generally not suitable for *teaching* children under five to sing. Most of them have a pitch range which is out of the average child's abilities as it requires too wide a tone-set of notes to be sung in tune. On top of that, many adults make the mistake of starting the melody at a pitch comfortable for the adult, but far too low for the child. When working with teachers I ask them to select a pitch which is comfortable for them and then count up five pitches before they start singing. Another mistake the untrained teacher can make is singing along with the children. Not only is it an excellent model for the teacher to listen to the children, and then the children to listen to the teacher, it also means that the teacher is able to assess who has found their singing voices.

When singing with the under fives you should sing complicated and interesting songs to them, in the same way that you would tell them a story. They love a game, actions, instructions and of course anticipation. I must stress here that hearing such a song does not mean that they should immediately attempt to sing it. We must first absorb what is too difficult for us and store it up for use as we develop.

When he starts singing, an average child needs to find his own voice first, and discover that he has a variety of voices: a talking voice, a whispering voice, a shouting voice (to be avoided due to damage to the vocal folds), a voice inside his head that I refer to as the 'thinking voice', and a singing voice, which uses quite different muscles from the other voices. Once a child has discovered his singing voice, it must be made very clear that a song is *sung*, whereas a verse is spoken. Both are valuable learning tools, but different.

'Have you brought your different voices?'

Once a child starts to sing in tune, the first interval I would start with would be the minor third. Singing is natural and the first singing sound a child makes is very often a falling minor third – which is like the sound of an old fashioned doorbell. 'Mummy', 'Daddy', 'Suzie' is a universal call, heard in playgrounds throughout the world.

Singing games should be started on a variety of pitches, higher and lower, involving just the interval of the minor third.

Hello   how are you?   Very   well   thank you.
(Ding-dong   ding-ding dong   ding-ding   dong   ding-dong)

Others that use just two pitches include.

- *Oh me, oh my, how I love my apple pie?*
- *Teddy bear, teddy bear, turn around.*
- *Hey, hey, look at me. I am happy, can't you see?*

These and many others can be found in *Growing with Music*, by Michael Stocks and Andrew Maddocks.[20]

Once a child can pitch-match a minor third in many different keys, the next natural interval is the major second that sits above the higher note, *la*.

Playground chants such as *I'm the king of the castle* lend themselves to this pattern.

The pentatonic scale leads on from these first few notes, leaving out the notoriously difficult minor second intervals that occur between the 3rd and the 4th of the scale and the 7th and 8th notes. (Very simply, the pentatonic scale is formed by using only the black notes on the piano.)

Remember children need to be listening to these intervals on a regular basis, but under the age of six, or even seven, they should not be expected to reproduce them accurately and should only be encouraged to do so if they can manage to find the interval with complete accuracy. If they can't, their muscles will learn to produce it incorrectly. In fact, it is true to say here that although correct practice may well make perfect, incorrect repetition (practice in effect), will make permanent, and the child may then, like the teenagers singing happy birthday, always sing out of tune, having practised and taught their muscles to produce incorrect pitches.

Another great asset to the learning brain is the ability to memorize song in any language, even using complete nonsense. Here is a pentatonic song that has been given new words in French by language teacher Sasha Baldwin, to help young children learn their body parts in that language.

épaules   jambes   pieds
épaules   jambes   pieds
tête   tête   épaules   jambes   genoux   pieds

so so   me   doh
épaules   jambes pieds
so so   me   doh
épaules   jambes pieds
la   la   so so   me   re re   doh
tête   tête   épaules jambes   genoux   pieds

Singing is a very important tool in the development of a young child. It teaches much more than music alone: listening, cooperation, taking turns, language skills, vocabulary, different languages, self-expression, internal thinking, diction, sequencing and structure, patterns and rhymes and communication. It is thought that singing makes you happier by causing endorphins to flow, helps you to breathe correctly, enhances your brain function and general wellbeing, teaches discipline, self-control, and in a group gives a sense of being part of a whole creative togetherness – which is fundamental to the wellbeing of the human spirit.

Why revive live singing, lullabies and nursery rhymes today?

In 2010 the government appointed Jean Gross, a former educational psychologist, to be a new 'communication champion'. She said that assessments of five-year-olds revealed that 18 per cent – over 100,000 – had fallen behind the expected level of speech development for their age:

> Middle-class children are struggling to learn how to talk because working parents are unable to offer them the quality time which is crucial to their speech development. They are often left in second-rate childcare and no longer benefit from the social inter-action of family mealtimes and bedtime stories [...] Fifty per cent of youngsters in some areas are starting formal schooling unable to link words together.[21]

A further impediment she identified was the trend for youngsters to spend time in front of machines such as TVs and computers instead of interacting with adults. She considers that one of the main contributory factors to this problem is the demise of conversation at home:

> Adults lead increasingly busy lives and many are not able to spend as much time talking to their children as generations before. Reading to your child is just as important as engaging in conversation, and the loss of a skill in one generation can be a lasting legacy to the next [...] If we have a generation who have not themselves been read to they are not going to do it when they

are parents. It's a ticking time bomb [...] Surveys suggest just 43 per cent of children are read to at bedtime [...] Pupils are starting primary school with a speaking age of just 18 months and an inability to form simple sentences.[22]

There are many reasons why speech and language problems exist or develop, many of which require professional assessment and intervention, but some of the increase in these problems in recent years stems directly from environmental factors which are entirely preventable. Talking, singing and reading with your child *every day* is one way of helping avoid many language problems developing later.

In a nutshell

- Speech and language begin with gesture and non-verbal utterances. In this sense, movement and music provide natural early language schooling.
- A mother's voice provides an acoustic link from pre-natal to post-natal life and is a child's first language teacher.
- Music and language share many elements in common. Language is musical and instrumental music is a form of language without words.
- Singing unites the verbal and non-verbal (musical) elements of language.
- Lullabies, nursery rhymes and songs prepare the infant ear and brain for the sounds of speech.
- Social interaction is vital for the development of reciprocal communication.
- 'Voicing' prepares the ground not only for speech but also for thinking in words.
- A child's own voice is one of the most powerful teaching instruments.
- Vibration provides multi-sensory stimulation affecting not only the body but also neuro-chemistry and emotions.
- Many children today are entering school with inadequate language ability.

Notes

1 C. Trevarthen: 'To be conscious: How infants' movements are planned, and how they engage with stimuli, things and people.' Paper presented at The 18th European Conference of Neuro-Developmental Delay in Children with Specific Learning Difficulties. Pisa, 23 September 2007.

2 C. Darwin: *The Expression of Emotions in Animals.* John Murray, London 1872.

3 P. Madaule: The ear-voice connection workshop. Chester, November 2001.

4 M. Lazarev: *Mamababy: Birth Before Birth.* Olma Media Group, Moscow 2007.

5 Ibid.

6 P. Eckerdal, B. Merker: 'Music and the action song in infant development: An interpretation.' Cited in Colwyn Trevarthen and Stephen Malloch (eds): *Communicative Musicality. Exploring the Basis of Human Companionship.* Oxford University Press 2009.

7 T. Stratford, A. Mera: 'The neurobiology of the therapeutic relationship between client and therapist: targeting symptomatic anxiety.' The 10th NPSA Congress. Paris, 20 June 2009.

8 Abba. Words from '*Thank you for the music.'* Popular song.

9 A. Berthoz: *The Brain's Sense of Movement.* Harvard University Press, Cambridge MA 2000.

10 R. Fisher: Personal communication 1993.

11 C. Lane: http://www.self-voice.com

12 P. Madaule: The ear-voice connection workshop seminar. Chester. November 2001.

13 A. Storr: *Music and the Mind.* Harper Collins, London 1993.

14 S.E. Shaywitz: 'Dyslexia.' Scientific American. November pp. 77–104, 1996.

15 A.D. Patel, E.J. Burnham: 'Music, language and grammatical processing.' Paper presented at the Symposium on: Music-Language Interactions in the Brain: From the Brainstem to Broca's Area. Presentation to The American Association for the Advancement of Science Conference. February 2010.

16 N. Kraus: 'Cognitive sensory interaction in the neural encoding of speech and music.' Paper presented at the Symposium on: Music-Language Interactions in the Brain: From the Brainstem to Broca's Area. Presentation to The American Association for the Advancement of Science Conference. February 2010.

17 Ibid.

18 Y. Schiftan: *The Missing Link. Musica Medica – Good Vibrations. A New Method of Multisensory Brain & Body Stimulation.* Unpublished, undated manuscript. Reproduced by permission of the author.

19 C. Lane: http://www.self-voice.com

20 Cambridge University Press, 1999.

21 J. Gross: Cited in 'Middle-class parents too busy to teach their children how to talk says "communications champion".' Laura Clark, *The Daily Mail,* 1 January 2010.

22 J. Gross: Cited in 'End of bedtime stories is wrecking children's speech warns government's new "communications champion".' Laura Clark, *The Daily Mail,* 16 October 2009.

CHAPTER 3

Lullabies, Carols and Nursery Rhymes

Lullabies

Mothers have sung to their children at bedtime to help lull or soothe them to sleep for generations. There are a number of theories about the origins of the word lullaby, one of which suggests that it describes the repetitive sounds mothers use when talking or singing to their babes such as *lully, lulla, lullay*, and *bye-bye*, or *bie* (also pronounced 'bye'), the latter describing generally soothing sounds such as running water or the whispering of the wind in the trees.

In classical music a lullaby is called a *berceuse* – a French word which means cradle song. Lullabies are usually in triple metre or 6/8 time, which has a characteristic swinging or rocking motion. Tonally berceuses are usually simple, often merely alternating tonic and dominant harmonies,* since the intended effect is to lull someone to sleep.

Lullabies are usually slow in pace, mimicking many of the movement experiences a baby has before birth. Slow motion is inclined to be soothing, while fast movement tends to arouse. The natural rhythms and pace of lullabies are therefore ideally suited for 'lulling' your baby to sleep.

---

* Tonic refers to keynote of the scale; dominant to the 5th note in the scale.

As mentioned in the 'Good vibrations' section in the previous chapter, children's response to live music is different from recorded music, and babies are particularly responsive when the music comes directly from the parent. The human interaction itself (touch, voice, and eye contact) is the important thing, using a form of language attuned to an infant's level of development, rather than the individual lullaby itself. However, all lullabies share a similar range of rhythms and tones – a form of universal language.

The peculiar structure of lullabies – like a story with a beginning, middle and end – appeals to children; and this pattern helps them learn structure and order, and exercise imagination:

> The melody and harmony are just intricate enough to stimulate the imagination slightly [...] yet also send an unspoken message of support and security, in a way no words can describe.[1]

Lullabies also help to strengthen the bond formed between parents and child before birth. In the mother's case this is through familiarity with her voice and movements – but the father also has a role. Michael Lazarev stresses the importance of introducing the father's voice to the unborn child through singing before birth. The mother, he says, is teacher, psychologist and doctor to her baby, but the father is assistant 'organizer of studies'.[2] Introducing father's voice also connects the child to a wider range of sound frequencies, and the process of singing lullabies not only influences the child's state but also that of the singing parent. This in itself may help to calm a child, who is likely to sense and react to the mood of a stressed parent.

Anyone can hum, chant or sing in some fashion. At the risk of repeating myself, it is really worth recognizing that your baby or infant will not judge your musical abilities. As far as she is concerned, you are the expert. A few tips may help to start a regular lullaby routine:

- Try to establish a regular bedtime routine that incorporates lullabies. Singing for as little as five minutes can be enough.
- Remembering the right words or singing in tune is not the important part. Warmth, meaning and security are conveyed

by the intimate resonance between you and the child, arising through the sound qualities you use and the emotional intent underlying them.

- Lazarev suggests developing your own lullabies before birth, using your baby's name if you have already chosen one. Lullabies can be created using the simplest words and music. For example, before birth:

Darling little (name of your baby),
I long to see your face,
I know your every movement
Hidden within this place.

After birth, the song can change:

Darling little (name of your baby),
Now I see your face
Small and round and perfect
Happy in this place.

When your baby is a little older you can introduce things from your everyday, shared experience, even things she may be a little scared of! For example, if your baby is afraid of dogs,

Hark, hark the dogs do bark
But (Charlie) *is safe in his bed,*
The silly dogs bark, chasing the dark
They only want to be fed!

- If you feel self-conscious singing alone, play a lullaby quietly on a CD in the background and sing along with it. Remember, it is *your* voice that matters.
- Gently rock or sway in time to the music. As your baby becomes drowsy, gradually reduce the amount of movement and simply hum to your child. Humming uses lower frequencies than singing and low frequencies tend to be more soporific. Allow yourself to become 'at one' with your baby and the music.

Many of the lullabies with which we are familiar today are thought to date from the seventeenth century onwards. The words of lullabies vary depending on historical period and region, but their basic form has been preserved and passed on through many generations. A few examples of traditional lullabies are given below.

Rock-a-Bye Baby

The most popular story about how 'Rock-a-bye Baby' came about is the American version about a pilgrim who came upon a Native American and saw the way she had suspended her baby from a tree in a birch-bark cradle. The idea was for the wind to sway the suspended cradle and rock the baby to sleep, but a branch might perhaps break, causing the cradle to fall.

Another story, from England, holds that 'Rock-a-bye Baby' refers to a family called the Kenyons who had a tree house in a huge yew tree. The Kenyon family had eight children and had hollowed out one of the boughs of the tree to be a cradle for the children. This yew tree was thought to be at least two thousand years old at the time.

'Rock-a-Bye Baby' in both sets of words shown below encourages gentle side-to-side rocking movements, which help soothe a baby to sleep.

Rock-a-bye Baby on the Tree Top

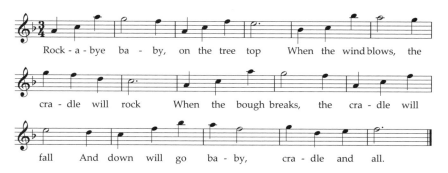

Rock-a-bye baby, on the tree top,
When the wind blows, the cradle will rock,
When the bough breaks, the cradle will fall
And down will go baby, cradle and all.

The second set of lyrics are found in a version of *Mother Goose*, published in 1916.

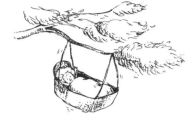

Rock-a-bye baby, the cradle is green
Father's a nobleman, mother's a queen
And Betty's a lady, and wears a gold ring
And Johnny's a drummer, and drums for
    the king.

Bye Baby Bunting

Both 'Bye Baby Bunting' and the 'Rocking Carol' are sung or said to a lilting, rocking rhythm.

In 'Bye Baby Bunting' the repetitive nature of the lines, the limited range of tones and the rhyming of words has a sleep inducing or 'hypnotic' effect (from the Greek word *hypnos* meaning sleep). The rhyming words 'bunting, hunting, milking, silking' also already prepares the very young child to distinguish minute differences in meaning between similar sounds.

Bye Baby Bunting

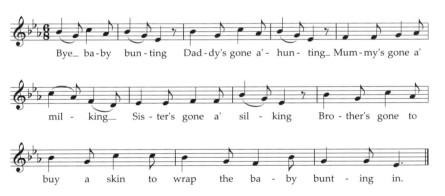

Bye baby bunting,
Daddy's gone a'hunting,
Mummy's gone a'milking,
Sister's gone a'silking,
Brother's gone to buy a skin
To wrap the baby bunting in.

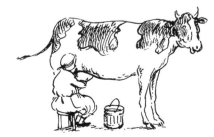

Rocking Carol

The Rocking Carol is of Czech origin. It was collected in the early 1920s and translated by Percy Dearmer for *The Oxford Book of Carols* in 1928. Dearmer was a clergyman and socialist with a keen interest in contemporary concerns who rescued neglected English carols and introduced European ones. The tune for the carol has a close resemblance to that of another traditional nursery rhyme, 'Twinkle, Twinkle, Little Star', and it is possible that this carol originally accompanied cradle rocking, a custom which began in German churches in medieval times and spread from there across Europe.[3]

Rocking Carol

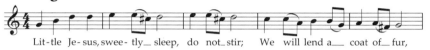

Lit-tle Je-sus, swee-tly_ sleep, do not_ stir; We will lend a__ coat of_ fur,

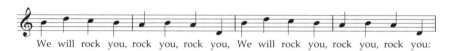

We will rock you, rock you, rock you, We will rock you, rock you, rock you:

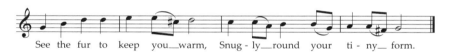

See the fur to keep you_warm, Snug-ly_round your ti-ny_ form.

Little Jesus, sweetly sleep, do not stir;
We will lend a coat of fur,
We will rock you, rock you, rock you,
We will rock you, rock you, rock you:
See the fur to keep you warm,
Snugly round your tiny form.

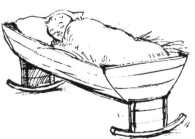

Mary's little baby, sleep, sweetly sleep,
Sleep in comfort, slumber deep;
We will rock you, rock you, rock you,
We will rock you, rock you, rock you:
We will serve you all we can,
Darling, darling little man.

Carols

The word carol comes from a Greek dance called a *choraulein,* which was accompanied by flute music and actually means dance, or a song of praise and joy.

Christmas carols are often several hundred years old, and while many of the oldest carols appear to originate from the Latin translation of the Bible, many older vernacular carols also survive. Some of the melodies that have survived are among the oldest types of music, having been passed on from generation to generation through singing and playing (oral tradition), whereas the words have changed over time. Many of the carols we are familiar with today, though, were actually written in the nineteenth and twentieth centuries, when the Victorians revived the tradition of celebrating Christmas.

Carols were first sung in Europe thousands of years ago, not as Christmas carols but as pagan songs, sung at the winter solstice celebrations (the shortest day of the year, 21 December) as people danced round stone circles.

In an attempt to make Christianity more appealing to potential converts, early Christians took over many of the pagan festivals, with Christmas replacing the pagan solstice celebrations, and new songs and forms of cerebration replacing the old. In the first thousand years of Christianity, 'carols' were sung to celebrate religious festivals, but the practice of celebrating Christmas declined during the Middle Ages.

In 1223 St. Francis of Assisi instigated a series of nativity plays in Italy. The plays featured songs or 'canticles' that told the story of the birth of Jesus and these became the ballads and 'musicals' of the time. They were particularly important in an age when most people were illiterate, books were rare and expensive items, and the Bible was written in Latin. The only way to teach people the Bible was through stories, songs, plays and images depicted in wall paintings and stained glass. Increasingly, canticles were sung in the local language so that the people watching the play could understand and join in, and many of these carols with a common story spread throughout Europe.

Many carols from the fifteenth century and the Elizabethan period are fables sung more for entertainment than as part of formal worship, although many are loosely based on the Christmas story. Travelling singers or minstrels would perform carols, often adapting the words to give them local relevance.

When the Puritans came to power in England in 1647, the celebrations and customs associated with former 'Papist' traditions were banned. A few carols survived to be resurrected in Victorian times by William Sandys and Davis Gilbert, who started to collect old Christmas music from villages in England.[4]

The Coventry Carol

This carol is based on the biblical story of the slaughter of the innocents by King Herod on hearing of the birth of a new king who he feared would grow up to challenge his authority.

The Coventry Carol was originally associated with English Mystery Plays, which have been traced back to 1456. Every year at the spring religious festival of Corpus Christi, the guilds of various towns would put on a series of plays illustrating Bible stories. At a time when the Roman Catholic Church refused to sanction Bibles in the vernacular, this was one of the few ways in which ordinary people could hear Bible stories. The Coventry Carol is one of the oldest surviving, unadapted carols, retaining both its original tune and words.

While such a brutal story seems a strange choice for singing a small baby to sleep, both the melody and the sound of words contain all the elements of the perfect lullaby, and the words of the story, like many fables, are a reminder that real life is brutal, bringing with it dangers as well as blessings. If for religious or ideological reasons you do not want to sing the words of the verses to your child, the melody and the refrain are enough.

The Coventry Carol

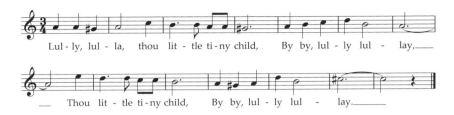

Lul - ly, lul - la, thou lit - tle ti -ny child, By by, lul - ly lul - lay,___

___ Thou lit - tle ti -ny child, By by, lul - ly lul - lay.___

Lully, lulla, thou little tiny child,
By by, lully lullay, thou little tiny child,
By by, lully lullay.

O sisters too, How may we do
For to preserve this day
This poor youngling,
For whom we do sing,
By by, lully lullay?

Lully, lulla, thou little tiny child,
By by, lully lullay, thou little tiny child,
By by, lully lullay.

Herod, the King, In his raging,
Charged he hath this day
His men of might,
In his own sight,
All young children to slay.

Lully, lulla, thou little tiny child,
By by, lully lullay, thou little tiny child,
By by, lully lullay.

That woe is me, Poor child for thee!
And ever morn and day,
For thy parting
Nor say nor sing
By by, lully lullay!

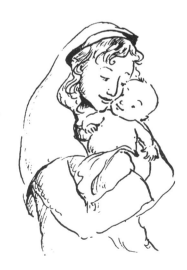

All Through the Night

Originally a Welsh nursery song, this lullaby sings of the fears and dreams of the night, promising the protection of tender love through the hours of darkness – for even as adults we tend to associate darkness with fear. The English lyrics are by Harold Boulton

Fear of the dark was described by Benedictine monk David Steindl-Rast[5] as a fear of 'no-thing-ness'. Born to live in a physical, material world, we tend to fear silence and empty spaces as confirmation of being alone. The most acute of the external senses – the sense of vision – is impaired in darkness, meaning we cannot use the things we normally see to help us find our way. In other words, there is no physical reference point in space.

Sleep brings with it separation from the outside world and from others, enclosing us in the inner world of the mind. It has sometimes been described as the little death.

In the monastic tradition, chants are sung during the canonical *hours*. *Hours* do not describe a unit of 60 minutes but *seasons* of the day, each having special features and opportunities. The first hour of the day is Vigils. Sung before the dawn breaks, Vigils 'is the night watch hour, the time for learning to trust the darkness', while Lauds greets the coming of the light and is a reminder of the gift that each new day brings. Compline completes the circle of the day making a transition into night and sleep, with prayer for 'a peaceful night and perfect end'. It finishes with a blessing and final hymn, similar to a mother singing her child to sleep.

Sleep, like darkness, also brings with it the opportunity for growth, restoration and healing. It opens a source of fresh beginning, of new ideas with which we can meet the challenges of the following day. We are born out of the darkness of the womb. Plants germinate and spread their first shoots in darkness under the ground, and the new buds of spring shoot from within the darkness and cold of winter. Although we may fear the dark, it is out of darkness that new life is born.

A mother's lullaby to her child is like a blessing and reassurance of love at the end of every day, an acknowledgement of the separation that will occur in sleep and an invitation to welcome sleep with all the benefits that it brings.

All Through the Night

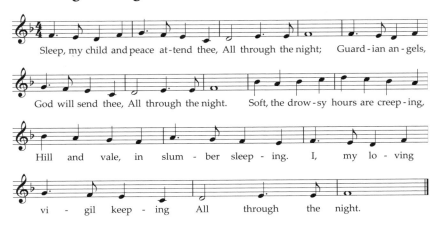

Sleep, my child and peace at-tend thee, All through the night; Guard-ian an-gels,
God will send thee, All through the night. Soft, the drow-sy hours are creep-ing,
Hill and vale, in slum - ber sleep - ing. I, my lo - ving
vi - gil keep - ing All through the night.

Sleep, my child and peace attend thee,
All through the night;
Guardian angels, God will send thee,
All through the night.

Soft, the drowsy hours are creeping,
Hill and vale, in slumber sleeping,
I, my loving vigil keeping
All through the night.

While the moon, her watch is keeping
All through the night;
While the weary world is sleeping
All through the night.

O'er thy spirit gently stealing
Visions of delight revealing,
Breathes a pure and holy feeling
All through the night.

Love to thee, my thoughts are turning
All through the night;
All for thee, my heart is yearning,
All through the night.

Though sad fate our lives may sever
Parting will not last forever,
There's a hope that leaves me never,
All through the night.

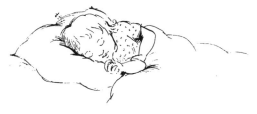

Brahms' Lullaby (Johannes Brahms)

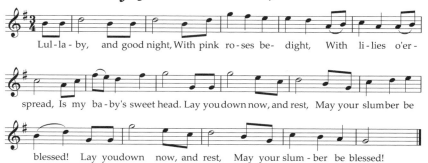

Lul-la-by, and good night, With pink ro-ses be-dight, With li-lies o'er-spread, Is my ba-by's sweet head. Lay you down now, and rest, May your slumber be blessed! Lay you down now, and rest, May your slum-ber be blessed!

Lullaby, and good night,
With pink roses bedight,
With lilies o'erspread,
Is my baby's sweet head.
Lay you down now, and rest,
May your slumber be blessed!
Lay you down now, and rest,
May thy slumber be blessed!

Lullaby, and good night,
You're your mother's delight,
Shining angels beside
My darling abide.
Soft and warm is your bed,
Close your eyes and rest your head.
Soft and warm is your bed,
Close your eyes and rest your head.

Sleepyhead, close your eyes.
Mother's right here beside you.
I'll protect you from harm,
You will wake in my arms.
Guardian angels are near,
So sleep on, with no fear.
Guardian angels are near,
So sleep on, with no fear.

Lullaby, and sleep tight.
Hush! My darling is sleeping,
On his sheets white as cream,
With his head full of dreams.
When the sky's bright with dawn,
He will wake in the morning.
When noontide warms the world,
He will frolic in the sun.

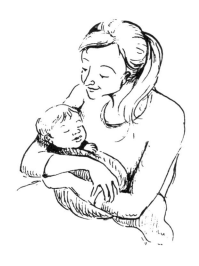

Hush, Little Baby

This is a traditional lullaby thought to be of American origin.

Mockingbirds are a group of New World passerine birds from the Mimidae family, which are best known for the habit of some species mimicking the songs of insect and amphibian sounds as well as other bird songs, often loudly and in rapid succession.

The repetitive nature of the tune with its answering phrase for each alternating line helps to keep a baby's attention, anticipating what will come next. The words promise all kinds of rewards to the baby if she is quiet, but lyrics can also be improvised if they remain within the overall rhythm and rhyme pattern. In this way the lullaby can be adapted to be special for each mother and child. For example:

And if that horse and cart fall down
Papa's gonna buy you a tumbling clown,
And if that clown don't you make you laugh
Papa's gonna buy you a sweet young calf,
And if that pretty little calf don't grow,
Papa's gonna buy you a bright pink bow …

Hush, Little Baby

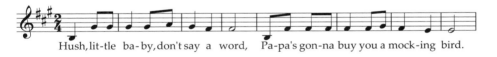

Hush, lit-tle ba-by, don't say a word, Pa-pa's gon-na buy you a mock-ing bird.

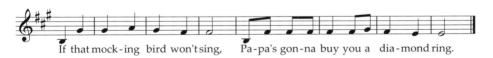

If that mock-ing bird won't sing, Pa-pa's gon-na buy you a dia-mond ring.

Hush, little baby, don't say a word,
Papa's gonna buy you a mockingbird.
And if that mockingbird won't sing,
Papa's gonna buy you a diamond ring.
And if that diamond ring turns to brass,
Papa's gonna buy you a looking glass.
And if that looking glass gets broke,
Papa's gonna buy you a billy goat.

And if that billy goat won't pull,
Papa's gonna buy you a cart and bull.
And if that cart and bull turn over,
Papa's gonna buy you a dog named Rover.
And if that dog named Rover won't bark,
Papa's gonna buy you a horse and cart.
And if that horse and cart fall down,
You'll still be the sweetest little baby in town.

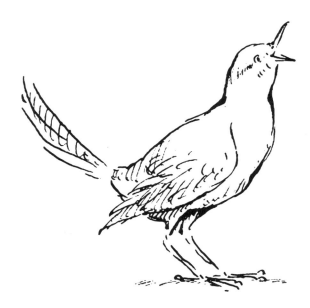

From lullabies to nursery rhymes

Nursery rhymes are traditionally sung or spoken to young children, but most were not originally designed for this purpose. Many reflect events in history and the political and social problems prevalent at the time and place where they developed, when outright criticism of authority would have resulted in punishment but allegory or parody were still possible. Many nursery rhymes originally played a rather similar role to today's political and social commentators, satirists and cartoonists. As such, they are an important part of a child's cultural history and heritage.

A few examples of well-known nursery rhymes for the very young to the pre-school child are included below to illustrate the continuing value and relevance of nursery rhymes for modern times.

For parents who would like a full anthology of nursery rhymes, there are many collections available, and the words of most well-known rhymes and their tunes can be found on the internet.

Twinkle, Twinkle, Little Star

The tune for this rhyme appears in many languages and is shared by other nursery rhymes such as 'Baa Baa Black Sheep' and the Alphabet Song. It is based on an original French melody 'Ah! vous dirai-je Maman'. Mozart and Dohnányi wrote a set of variations on the tune; and Saint-Saëns used the melody for one movement of his suite for children, 'Carnival of the Animals'.

Like many nursery rhymes, the original French version 'Ah! vous dirai-je, Maman' is a story far more suitable for adults, in which a girl confides to her mother that she has been seduced by Silvandre and is beaten by 'L'amour'. The more innocent English rhyme was originally written as a poem, 'The Star', by the sisters Ann and Jane Taylor in the early nineteenth century and published in *Rhymes for the Nursery* in London in 1806.[6]

Young children are fascinated by light, their visual attention being drawn towards anything that shines lighter, brighter or moves within their visual field in the first weeks of life. The human eye has a remarkable capacity to detect a single source of light in the dark. In theory, in a typical dark sky, the dark-adapted human eye has the ability to see several thousand of the brightest stars. In perfect dark sky conditions about 45,000 stars brighter than $+8^m$ might be visible.[7] In practice this ability is affected by surrounding light pollution, reducing the number actually visible in a modern city centre to between 200 and 400. This is one of the reasons why, when we travel to remoter parts of the world, we are often struck by the multitude and brilliance of stars in the night sky, and can once again see them with something like a young child's wonder.

Introducing your child to this well-known tune at an early age will later allow its familiarity to be built on when learning the alphabet. The child can also later rediscover this tune in more intricate and complex forms, as used by a number of classical composers. At every stage in life we are able to learn and remember something new more easily when we can 'attach' it to something already known. Familiarizing children with these simple and timeless melodies from an early age means they are better able to recognize and memorize new material with related themes.

Twinkle, Twinkle, Little Star

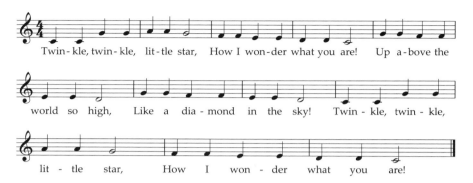

Twin-kle, twin-kle, lit-tle star, How I won-der what you are! Up a-bove the world so high, Like a dia-mond in the sky! Twin-kle, twin-kle, lit-tle star, How I won-der what you are!

Twinkle, twinkle, little star,
How I wonder what you are!
Up above the world so high,
Like a diamond in the sky!

Chorus
Twinkle, twinkle, little star,
How I wonder what you are!

When the blazing sun is gone,
When he nothing shines upon,
Then you show your little light,
Twinkle, twinkle, all the night.

(repeat chorus)

Then the traveller in the dark,
Thanks you for your tiny spark,
He could not see which way to go,
If you did not twinkle so.

(repeat chorus)

In the dark blue sky you keep,
And often through my curtains peep,
For you never shut your eye,
Till the sun is in the sky.

(repeat chorus)

As your bright and tiny spark,
Lights the traveller in the dark –
Though I know not what you are,
Twinkle, twinkle, little star.

(repeat chorus)

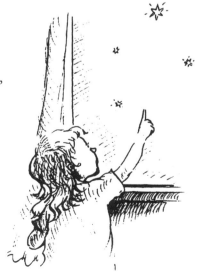

Baa Baa Black Sheep

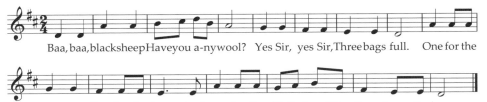

This rhyme dates back to 1272 when Edward I imposed an export tax on wool. One-third of income derived from wool went to the king (the 'master') and one-third to the local feudal lord (referred to as the 'dame'), leaving a third for the farmer (the 'little boy who lives down the lane').

Payment was made in sacks of wool. At the time, wool from a black sheep was worth less than ordinary wool, probably because it involved a more complicated dyeing process.

The problem of taxation changes little from one generation to the next, and in this sense the rhyme is as apt for children today as it was 900 years ago. However, once again it is the alliterative* features of the rhyme 'Baa, baa, black …' and, imitation of some of the first sounds made by babies of all cultures which has made it an enduring favourite.

In recent years it has been the subject of controversy in the United Kingdom by some people who suggest it has racial connotations. When seen in its historical context, this is an entirely erroneous interpretation, and changing the words to 'Baa, baa, rainbow sheep' belittles the rhyme's musical, onomatopoeic and linguistic developmental value for young children.

Baa, Baa, Black Sheep

Baa, baa, black sheep Have you a-ny wool? Yes Sir, yes Sir, Three bags full. One for the

ma-ster One for the dame, And one for the lit-tle boy Who lives down the lane.

Baa, baa, black sheep,	One for the master,
Have you any wool?	One for the dame,
Yes Sir, yes Sir,	And one for the little boy
Three bags full.	Who lives down the lane.

---

* Alliteration describes a literary or rhetorical stylistic device that consists of repeating the same consonant sound at the beginning of two or more words in close succession. An example is the tongue-twister, 'Peter Piper picked a peck of pickled peppers'.

Ring-a-Ring-a-Roses

This rhyme first appeared in published form in Kate Greenaway's *Mother Goose* in 1881, much later than the popular belief that it originated from the time of the Black Death in the 1340s or the Great Plague of London in 1665–6. The theory was that the 'ring' referred to the ring of sores around the mouths of plague victims, and the 'a-tishoo' imitated the sneezing that accompanied the disease. Kate Greenaway's version uses the words 'Hush! hush! hush! hush' while other versions use 'a-tishoo, a-tishoo'.

Whatever its true origin, the rhyme contains all the features needed to capture the young child's attention: rhyme, repetition and alliteration; and actions to accompany the song.

One of the first things a child must master is control of her body in a gravity-determined environment. The sense of balance precedes and facilitates our capacity to move, and responds to stimulus in three planes of movement:

1   Rotation around a vertical axis (spinning, carousels, etc.)
2   Rotation through a horizontal axis (rolling and rocking forwards and backwards, swings, see-saws, etc.)
3   Side-to-side tilting movements and up and down movements.

Children gain control of their body in space through movement experience of each of these planes of motion. 'Ring-a-Ring-a-Roses' encourages movement around the vertical axis, helping to train one part of the balance apparatus to improve control of the body, as well as other centres which need to cooperate with balance. Other songs such as 'Here We Go Round the Mulberry Bush' encourage the same movement activity. 'Ring-a-Ring-a-Roses' also teaches children how to fall down and get up again. The first lesson in learning control of balance is learning to fall and get up – and then learning how not to fall again.[8]

Ring-a-Ring-a-Roses

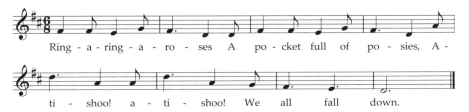

Ring - a - ring - a - ro - ses A po - cket full of po - sies, A - ti - shoo! a - ti - shoo! We all fall down.

Ring-a-ring-a-roses,
A pocket full of posies;
Hush! hush! hush! hush!
We're all tumbled down.

or

Ring a-ring o' roses,
A pocketful of posies.
A-tishoo! a-tishoo!
We all fall down.

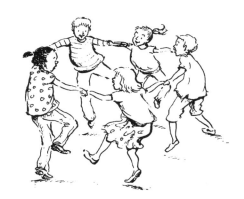

Hey Diddle Diddle

This somewhat surreal rhyme is a riot for the imagination, invoking images of logically impossible events (though perfectly possible in the young child's fantasy world, as yet unrestricted by natural or scientific laws).

The young child's visual world is limited by her height and movement capabilities. This means that objects insignificant to adults have proportionally much greater significance to the young child. When sitting in a high chair for example, the dish and the spoon are very important objects; a cow in the field is a huge monster, and there is no reason why, before understanding of distance and perspective develop, this large creature should not be able to jump over the distant, tiny moon.

Hey Diddle Diddle is a wonderful example of the mixture of rhyme, alliteration, fantasy and fun which are the hallmarks of enduring childhood songs. The term 'Hey diddle diddle' was originally a colloquialism used in much the same way as 'hey nonny no' – which can be found in traditional British folksongs.[9]

Hey Diddle Diddle

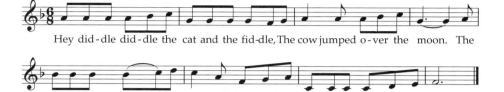

Hey did-dle did-dle the cat and the fid-dle, The cow jumped o-ver the moon. The
lit-tle dog laughed to see such fun And the dish ran a-way with the spoon!

Hey diddle diddle, the cat and the fiddle,
The cow jumped over the moon.
The little dog laughed to see such fun
And the dish ran away with the spoon!

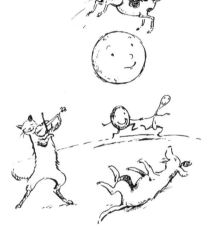

Jack and Jill

This rhyme is thought to originate from the French Revolution when, during the reign of terror in 1793, Louis XVI (Jack) was deprived of his head (crown) at the guillotine, followed by the queen, Marie Antoinette (Jill). At times of social and political unrest, it is often not safe to discuss political events openly, but they can be referred to in story, rhyme and jest. The second verse allows for a happy ending. Vinegar was relevant because it has powerful antiseptic properties for treating bumps and wounds.

The spelling and words of nursery rhymes change over generations as for a long time they were passed on by word of mouth. However, they also change to fit the political and social needs of the time, hence our somewhat updated version of 'Jack and Jill' which takes political correctness and modern health concerns into account!

Jack and Jill

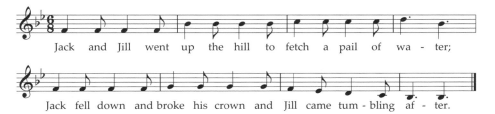

Jack and Jill went up the hill to fetch a pail of wa - ter;

Jack fell down and broke his crown and Jill came tum - bling af - ter.

Jack and Jill went up the hill to fetch a pail of water;
Jack fell down and broke his crown,
And Jill came tumbling after.

Up got Jack, and home did trot
As fast as he could caper.
He went to bed and bound his head
With vinegar and brown paper.

Jack and Jill – the modern version

Jack and Jill went into town
To fetch some chips and sweeties.
He can't keep his heart rate down,
And she's got diabetes.

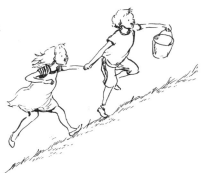

Humpty Dumpty

In the fifteenth century, Humpty Dumpty was the colloquial term to describe someone fat. It was also the name given to an extremely large canon situated on the wall of St. Mary's Wall Church in Colchester, designed to defend the Parliamentarian town of Colchester during the English Civil War (1642–49). However, Colchester temporarily fell into the hands of the Royalists and canon fire from the expelled Parliamentarians damaged the wall, bringing Humpty Dumpty to the ground. When the Royalists tried to restore Humpty Dumpty to an elevated firing position, 'not all the King's horses and all the King's men could put Humpty Dumpty together again'. Colchester eventually fell to the Parliamentarians after a siege lasting several weeks.

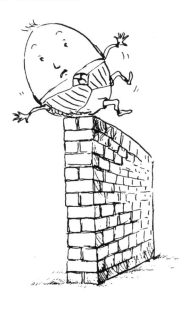

Modern illustrations for this rhyme usually depict Humpty Dumpty as a large egg, dressed as a rotund man. As a young child I always thought the rhyme was a moral tale to explain that something which was brittle on the outside could be easily broken and impossible to put back together again. I could never see a boiled egg for breakfast without thinking of Humpty Dumpty, and the habit, common when I was a child, of putting a knitted hat on a boiled egg to keep it warm, and drawing a face on the egg, reinforced the image.

'Imagination' describes the ability to form 'images in the brain' or mental images. Any nursery rhyme, song or story which encourages children to form mental images helps to develop the vocabulary for creative thinking, because complex ideas come not just from words but from images, sensations and experience which come together in a new form. It was once said that genius is not the creation of something completely new, but rather new connections of knowledge and experience in a mind that is open and ready to see in new ways.

This is why songs, rhymes and the telling of stories are still so vital in childhood. When children listen and form mental images from what they hear, they make new connections. When sound

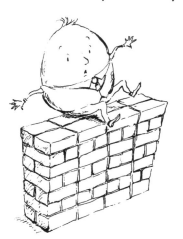

and image are presented together, as in television or electronic games, the creative process of translating what is heard into a mental image is bypassed. It has already been done by the creators of the programme who have predetermined what the child should 'see'.

The processes of translating sounds into mental images and vice-versa will be needed a few years later when a child learns to read and write. Reading involves matching a series of visual symbols on the page to the *sounds* of letters and words; writing involves the translation of thoughts 'heard' inside the head into visual symbols, or ideas seen as mental images into speech sounds which must then be translated into visual symbols. These are highly complex neurological processes involving communication between the two sides of the brain in *both* directions (from left to right and from right to left), as well as the matching of information derived from different sensory systems.

The simple practice of singing, telling stories and reading to your child lays the foundations for these complex skills.

One of the 'modern' versions of the rhyme may entertain adults, though it does not have quite the same ring for children!

Humpty Dumpty

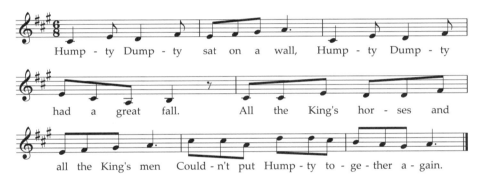

Humpty Dumpty sat on a wall,
Humpty Dumpty had a great fall.
All the King's horses, and all the King's men
Couldn't put Humpty together again!

Humpty Dumpty – the modern version

Humpty Dumpty sat on a wall,
Humpty Dumpty had a great fall.
The structure of the wall was incorrect,
So he won a grand with Claims Direct!

Rhymes for older children (aged 3–6)

The Owl and the Pussycat, by Edward Lear

Edward Lear's 'nonsense' rhymes provide a marvellous example of 'the music of language'[10] and the way in which this can convey the most powerful human emotions. A young child may not understand the concept of adult romantic love but it does understand longing, joy and the sensuous delights suggested by 'dining on mince and slices of quince' and the freedom of being 'hand in hand on the edge of the sand' as 'they danced by light of the moon'.

When adults fall in love they summon the joys and longings of childhood from the deeper reaches of the soul, awakening all childhood's sensory experiences and revisiting them together as a part of the process of attachment.

It is not necessary for the young child to understand the meaning of every word. Meaning is implicit in the music and metaphor of the language. At the same time, the use of more advanced language helps to extend the young child's vocabulary. *A beautiful pea green boat* immediately invokes images of the colour of the boat, while *you elegant fowl* is clearly intended as a compliment but at the same time describes the species to which the recipient belongs. Children who are fortunate enough to grow up surrounded by adults with a rich vocabulary naturally absorb implicit language complexities through listening and conversation that others may be deprived of. This is not necessarily a matter of education or class. A rich and vivid vernacular exists in many walks of life, and is often particularly developed in people living close to the land and nature in rural communities.

Chapter 2 stressed the importance of a mother's voice. Research has indicated that hearing the sound of the mother's voice is as good as receiving a cuddle. It releases a hormone involved in love and attachment (oxytocin) and reduces stress levels in the child. The reading of poems and telling of stories uses this powerful instrument of comfort and attachment as well as introducing the child to new vocabulary, stories and ideas.[11]

The Owl and the Pussycat

The Owl and the Pussy-cat went to sea
   In a beautiful pea green boat,
They took some honey, and plenty of money,
   Wrapped up in a five pound note.
The Owl looked up to the stars above,
   And sang to a small guitar,
'O lovely Pussy! O Pussy my love,
   What a beautiful Pussy you are,
     You are,
     You are!
What a beautiful Pussy you are!'

Pussy said to the Owl, 'You elegant fowl!
   How charmingly sweet you sing!
O let us be married! Too long we have tarried:
   But what shall we do for a ring?'
They sailed away, for a year and a day,
   To the land where the Bong-tree grows
And there in a wood a Piggy-wig stood
   With a ring at the end of his nose,
     His nose,
     His nose,
With a ring at the end of his nose.

'Dear pig, are you willing to sell for one shilling
   Your ring?' Said the Piggy, 'I will.'
So they took it away, and were married next day
   By the Turkey who lives on the hill.
They dined on mince, and slices of quince,
   Which they ate with a runcible spoon;
And hand in hand, on the edge of the sand,
   They danced by the light of the moon,
     The moon,
     The moon,
They danced by the light of the moon.

Games for mother, father and baby

Pat-a-Cake, Pat-a-Cake

Probably originating in the weekly task of baking and icing in the kitchen, this rhyme is always accompanied by a hand-clapping game and is suitable for children from about 9 months; but much older children continue to enjoy it, and it can be made more complicated for older children. Hand clapping between adult and child helps to develop hand-eye coordination, use of one hand at a time and the ability to cross the midline. It also helps to inhibit any remaining traces of the infant grasp reflex which can interfere with the development of finger and thumb opposition movements necessary for fine motor tasks (particularly writing), if it remains active for too long. As the game becomes more complex it helps to develop sequential memory through the pattern of the game.

In a study which examined the impact of hand-clapping songs on children in kindergarten and the first grades, researchers found that, 'children who sing these songs demonstrate skills absent in children who don't take part in similar activities […] children who spontaneously perform hand-clapping songs in the yard have neater handwriting, write better and make fewer spelling errors'.[12]

Pat-a-Cake, Pat-a-Cake

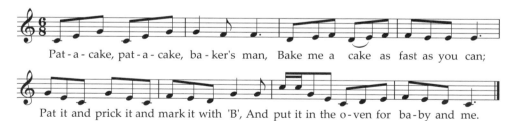

Pat-a-cake, pat-a-cake, ba-ker's man, Bake me a cake as fast as you can;

Pat it and prick it and mark it with 'B', And put it in the o-ven for ba-by and me.

Pat-a-cake, pat-a-cake, baker's man
Bake me a cake as fast as you can;
Pat it and prick it and mark it with 'B',
And put it in the oven for baby and me.

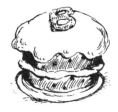

Round and Round the Garden

This game can be played with babies once they are able to sit up. Gently stroking the palm of the baby's hand using a circular motion while saying 'round and round', then moving in small steps up the lower arm to 'one step, two step', and finally tickling under the arm pit. Under 9 months, the baby may close his fingers over the adult's finger in a palmar grasp, but this will gradually modify as he is able to open his fingers and actively seek to be stroked.

Round and Round the Garden

Round and round the garden
Like a teddy bear.
One step, two step,
Tickle you under there.

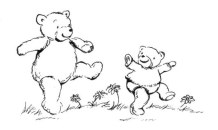

Down in the Deep Blue Sea

This is a game played with the child sitting on the parent's knee facing the parent.

First the child is gently bounced on the knee and the parent gradually allows the knees to part.

During the first line, the child is lowered a little way between the parent's knees and then lifted up again.

At the second line the child is lowered further and then pulled up.

At the words, 'down, down, down, down', the child is dropped progressively lower, but not does not quite touch the floor.

On the final line, the child is dropped as low as possible and held there for a few seconds before being pulled all the way up again.

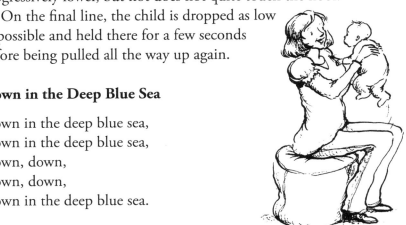

Down in the Deep Blue Sea

Down in the deep blue sea,
Down in the deep blue sea,
Down, down,
Down, down,
Down in the deep blue sea.

This is the Way the Ladies Ride

This is another game played sitting on the parent's knee facing the parent, and holding the parent's two hands. The parent starts to make gentle up and down jogging movements with the knees, consistent with the demure and gentle ride of a lady wearing a long dress. As the rhyme progresses, so the movements become more vigorous, until the farmer's ride is really bumpy and the child has to hold on to the parent's hands to avoid falling off the knee.

The movements should be tailored to your child's personal level of enjoyment, and if you have a physically timid child, tone down the robustness of the final movements so that your child is not frightened.

In another version, a plough boy does actually tumble off the horse and land in a ditch, with much hilarity for slightly older children (four to six).

This is the Way the Ladies Ride

This is the way the ladies ride,
Trit trot, trit trot.
This is the way the ladies ride,
Trit trot, trit trot. Trit trot.

This is the way the gentlemen ride,
A gallop, a trot, a gallop, a trot.
This is the way the gentlemen ride,
A gallop, a trot, a gallop.

This is the way the farmer rides
Jiggety-jog, jiggety-jog,
This is the way the farmer rides,
Jiggety-jiggety-jog.

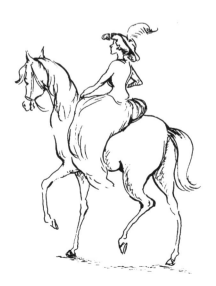

Here We Go Round the Mulberry Bush

The rhyme was first recorded in the mid-nineteenth century by James Orchard Halliwell, who suggested the original words might have been 'Here we go round the bramble bush'. The song and associated actions are traditional, and have parallels in several other European countries – although the type of bush used in the rhyme may vary regionally.

The words and game can be extended to include all sorts of different daily activities, and original verses can be updated: sweeping the floor, can be followed, for example, by 'This is the way we vacuum the floor' etc. Personally, I think the traditional rhyme should always be used first as it provides a reminder of archetypal activities, rhythms and gestures in domestic life before technology provided the many labour-saving devices we have come to depend on today. Monday was traditionally the day for washing; it would be put out to dry in the fresh air if the weather was fine, or draped over a pulley or indoor washing line if it was wet. A whole day was needed to air the washing before it was ready to be ironed, hence Tuesday was the traditional day for ironing. Floors had to be swept and all crumbs and debris removed before it was ready for washing and scrubbing. These simple rhymes and actions help the young child to learn that there is a sequence in how things are done, as well as building sequential memory for the order of the days of the week.

I was reminded of how powerful the combination of song and action is for developing vocabulary when visiting a Steiner School in London and being invited to observe a German language lesson. The entire lesson was based on a song that the children had learned by rote about the parts of the body, associated sensations and responses – such as itching and scratching, thirst and drinking; and spatial relationships such as: tall and short, big and little, narrow and wide. Young children, who had not yet learned to read or write, understood the German words for names and actions, nouns and verbs as if German was their first language. They were in fact learning a second language in the same way one learns a mother tongue: through seeing, hearing, acting and vocalizing; and by linking what is felt through the senses to specific speech sounds.

Here We Go Round the Mulberry Bush

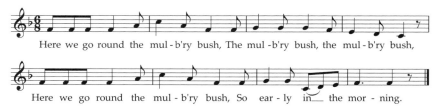

Here we go round the mul-b'ry bush, The mul-b'ry bush, the mul-b'ry bush,

Here we go round the mul-b'ry bush, So ear-ly in the mor-ning.

Here we go round the mulberry bush
The mulberry bush, the mulberry bush
Here we go round the mulberry bush
So early in the morning.

This is the way we wash our clothes
Wash our clothes, wash our clothes
This is the way we wash our clothes
So early Monday morning.

This is the way we iron our clothes
Iron our clothes, iron our clothes
This is the way we iron our clothes
So early Tuesday morning.

This is the way we mend our clothes
Mend our clothes, mend our clothes
This is the way we mend our clothes
So early Wednesday morning.

This is the way we sweep the floor
Sweep the floor, sweep the floor
This is the way we sweep the floor
So early Thursday morning.

This is the way we scrub the floor
Scrub the floor, scrub the floor
This is the way we scrub the floor
So early Friday morning.

This is the way we bake our bread
Bake our bread, bake our bread
This is the way we bake our bread
So early Saturday morning.

This is the way we go to church
Go to church, go to church
This is the way we go to church
So early Sunday morning.

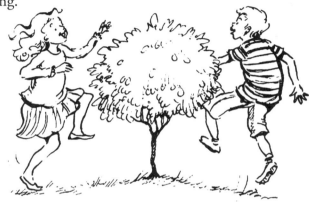

Notes

1 T. Thompson, cited in article 'Say Goodnight to Sleepless Nights with Lullabies' by Sarah Molnar. http://www.curiousparents.

2 M. Lazarev: *Mammababy: Birth Before Birth*. Olma Media Group, Moscow 2007.

3 http://www.hymnsandcarolsofchristmas.com/Hymns_and_Carols/rocking_carol-2.htm

4 Suite101: Medieval Christmas Carols pt. 1: Origins http://medievalhistory.suite101.com/article.cfm/medieval_christmas_carols_pt__1#ixzz0gv8Q8B3C

5 D. Steindl-Rast: *The Music of Silence*. Harper, San Francisco 1995.

6 J. and A. Taylor: *Rhymes for the Nursery* 1806.

7 John E. Bortle: 'The Bortle Dark-Sky Scale'. Sky & Telescope. http://www.skyandtelescope.com/resources/darksky/3304011.html. February 2001.

8 O. Schrager: 'Balance control, age and language development.' Paper presented at the 12th European Conference of Neuro-Developmental Delay in Children with Specific Learning Difficulties. Chester, March 2000.

9 http://www.famousquotes.me.uk/nursery_rhymes/hey_diddle_diddle.htm

10 S.A. Goddard Blythe: *The Well-Balanced Child*. Hawthorn Press, Stroud 2002

11 'For comfort, mom's voice works as well as a hug.' ScienceDaily.com. Science News www.sciencedaily.com. 12 May 2010.

12 American Associates, Ben-Gurion University of the Negev. 'Hand-clapping songs improve motor and cognitive skills, research shows.' Science Daily. 3/5/2010. www.sciencedaily.com.2010/04/100428090954.htm

CHAPTER 4

More Action Songs and Rhymes for Babies to Preschoolers

by Jane Williams (PhD)

Illustrations by Tom Kerr

Dr Jane Williams, who contributed this chapter, is a director of Toddler Kindy GymbaROO in Australia. There is a little overlap here with some material elsewhere in the book, but we felt that repetition was no bad thing!

GymbaROO (also known as KindyROO in Europe and Asia) is a programme combining parent/carer education with play. It was started more than thirty years ago by Margaret Sassé who also co-founded ANSUA – A New Start for the Under Achiever – in Melbourne. ANSUA focused on helping children who were struggling with learning at school, and after ten years of working with children with problems, Margaret Sassé realized that many of the difficulties faced by older children could have been picked up and corrected when they were younger.

In 1982, Toddler Kindy GymbaROO was launched as a preventative parent education and fun learning centre specializing in nurturing child development from 6 weeks to 5 years of age. GymbaROO/ KindyROO provides a fun-filled platform for parents and carers to gain greater knowledge of children's developmental needs and natural ways in which to maximise their child's development. This is so much more important in today's world, where modern life has de-naturalized the environmental stimuli that optimize the brain's potential. GymbaROO/KindyROO now performs the function of helping parents to put these natural stimuli back into their children's everyday life in a fun and enjoyable way, and to understand why this is important. Today, over 30,000 families in Australasia attend the programme every week. The GymbaROO/KindyROO website www.gymbaroo.com.au explains that:

> Children are developing 24/7 and not just for the 45 minutes a week they spend at GymbaROO, so what we really try to do is provide parents/carers with activities that can be done at home for the rest of the week. It is not just about providing activities, but also 'how and why' those activities help the brain develop. We have a different hand-out every week for each age-related development group. All teachers must be tertiary qualified (school teachers, nurses, occupational or physical therapists) before even being accepted for GymbaROO training; they need to learn and understand all about neuro-physiological development and then be able to communicate this to you little by little – as you need it. We also explore important issues such as balance, posture and motor development, as well as their importance to overall development.

While some of the nursery rhymes and games featured in this chapter were introduced in the last chapter, here they are developed further or in slightly different ways as action games. Children can first be introduced to the music and words at an early age as lullabies and nursery rhymes, and then explore familiar tunes and rhymes again in more robust and active ways through action games as they grow in strength and develop. This process of introducing new challenges to familiar patterns – known as 'layered' learning – encourages integration of learning pathways in the brain.

Babies – non-mobile

In all cultures, as we saw, parents instinctively communicate with infants in a musical manner, using a wide range of sing-song-like phrases ('motherese'). Parents find that their babies respond very positively to such communication, in fact, babies actually encourage it by rewarding the parents with smiling, lighting up their eyes, gurgling and paying close attention to the face of the singer.

Amazingly babies not only recognize different tunes, but can also differentiate between changes in musical notes, as well as between tones. Babies also notice changes in tempo, the speed at which the music is played, and rhythm.

Rhythmical activities to share with your baby

- Begin by introducing your young baby to music by playing soothing music quietly in his room. Classical music has been found to stimulate the brain, especially music by Mozart, Vivaldi, and music from the Baroque period. However, where possible live music is always best since it is not artificially mediated as electronic vibration.
- Sing nursery rhymes with your baby. Repeat the same rhymes regularly.
- Massage your baby while playing music or singing to him, stroking in time to the music.
- Tickling rhymes are a must. 'Round and Round the Garden' is a familiar one to start with (see below).
- Vary the tone of your voice when talking to your baby: talk, hum, sing and chant (especially rhymes and poems) during changing, feeding etc.
- Introduce new songs that have different rhythms. Baby will begin to recognize the faster or slower beat.
- Singing can be done with movement from three months or earlier. Start by rocking or swaying your infant while playing a piece of music, singing a rhyme or saying a poem. Lay the baby across your lap and bob your knees gently up and down, or rock sideways. Bouncing activities such as 'Ride a Cock horse' (see below) begin to introduce the 'beat' of the music.

Massage rhymes

Massage is a very important way of helping your baby learn about his body. It also makes both baby and parents feel calm and relaxed. The health benefits of regular massage cannot be overestimated! For these massage poems, you do not need to sing, but use a melodious voice so the baby hears the rhythm of the words *and* feels the rhythm of the movement as you stroke, tickle or squeeze your baby's body.

Here's Your Head (GymbaROO)

Here's your head, let's stroke your hair, *Lie baby on back, stroke baby's head*
Tap your cheeks and tickle your ears. *Tap cheeks, tickle ears*
Rub your shoulders, stroke your sides, *Rub shoulders*
Tap your chest and hide your eyes. *Tap chest, hide eyes with your hands*
Peek-a-boo *Open hands and look into your baby's eyes!*

Stroke your ribs right round to the back, *Stroke ribs*
Tickle your tummy and tap on your back. *Tickle tummy and tap the back*
Go down your arms, your legs and your feet, *Run hands down legs and feet*
Now squash you up so your head meets your feet. *Raise feet and legs to touch his nose*

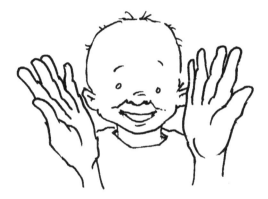

Pease Porridge Hot

This traditional rhyme has a great beat. Tap on your baby's body while chanting the words.

Pease porridge hot, *Tap baby's feet*
Pease porridge cold, *Tap baby's legs*
Pease porridge in the pot *Tap baby's back or tummy*
Nine days old. *Tap baby's chest*
Some like it hot, *Tap baby's hands*
Some like it cold, *Tap baby's arms*
Some like it in the pot *Tap baby's chest*
Nine days old. *Gently tap baby's head*

Rain

Rain on the grass,	*Tap fingers on baby's feet*
Rain on the trees,	*Tap fingers on baby's arms*
Rain on the rooftop,	*Tap fingers on baby's head*
But not on me!	
Rain on the grass,	*Tap fingers on feet*
Rain on the trees,	*Tap fingers on legs*
Rain on the windows,	*Tap fingers on face*
But not on me.	*Give baby a hug!*

Round and Round the Garden

The ever popular 'tickling' rhyme is loved by all age groups – not just babies! The youngest babies will not yet be opening the palm of their hands, so you can tickle on the back of the hand, on the feet – in fact on any exposed body part at all! Massaging bare skin is very stimulating to the sense of touch and helps your baby learn about his own body. Using a rhyme while tickling helps your baby learn about rhythm and how there are different sections that involve different responses.

Round and round the garden	*Use your fingers to tickle baby's hand, feet or body*
Like a teddy bear	
One step, two step	*Step fingers up the arm/leg or chest*
Tickle you under there.	*Tickle under the arm pit*

… and some variations …

Round and round the garden	*Repeat above but use a different body part!*
Like a little mouse	
One step, two step	
In his little house.	

Round and round the garden
Like a garden gnome
One step, two step
Can you find his home?

These are Baby's Fingers

These are baby's fingers	*Stroke or tickle baby's hands*
These are baby's toes	*Stroke or tickle baby's toes*
This is baby's belly button	*Tickle around the belly button*
Round and round it goes.	

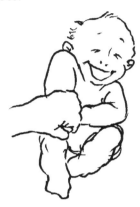

I Hear Thunder

Babies have little idea about where their body starts and ends. This is a fun rhyme that increases body awareness through different types of touch and sound.

I hear thunder	
I hear thunder	*Loud tapping on floor or tap on baby's body*
Hark don't you?	*Whisper*
Hark don't you?	
Pitter patter raindrops	*Wriggle fingers down and touch baby*
Pitter patter raindrops	
I'm wet through, so are you.	*(Loud) hug self and then baby*

Action songs

Action songs help a baby learn about his body. These fun tunes help you introduce your baby to his different body parts while you sing and move them in different ways. Learning that they have arms and legs and a tummy is important to help babies gain control over their movements. You will need to assist your baby to move his body as he is not yet able to do these actions by himself.

Mirror Song (GymbaROO)

This is a really great activity if your baby is not keen on tummy time and you wish to encourage greater enjoyment of this important position! Lie baby down in front of a mirror. If your baby is not settled, you can lie down next to your baby as well. Sing to the tune of 'Where is Thumbkin?' below.

Where is baby?
Where is baby?
Here she is!
Here she is!
How are you today *(name)*
Very well, I thank you
Stay and play
Stay and play. *(clap)*

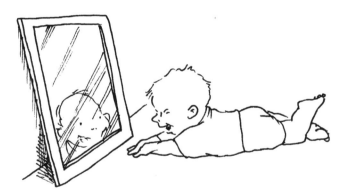

Body Moves (to the tune of 'The Bear Went Over the Mountain')

My arms are starting to wiggle, *wiggle your baby's arms etc*
My arms are starting to wiggle,
My arms are starting to wiggle,
Around and around and around.
My legs are starting to wiggle …
My tummy's starting to tickle …
etc.

Open Up My Arms Out Wide (GymbaROO)

Open up my arms out wide	*Open arms out wide*
Bring them back, right to my side	*Bring arms in to side*
Lift my left arm and then my right	*Lift one arm up and then other arm up*
Cuddle them across my chest so tight	*Cross arms over chest*
Kick my legs, up, down, up, down	*Kick legs up and down*
Roll my hips – round and around	*Hold hips and roll on the spot*
Now bump my knees – tap, tap, tap	*Bump knees together*
And rub my feet upon the mat.	*Rub feet on the mat*

Bicycle

I'm riding my bicycle all over town	*Pedal baby's legs, first slowly,*
First very slowly	*then quickly*
Then fast, round and round!	

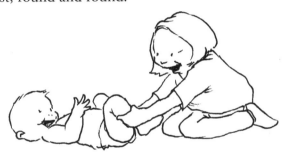

We're Rolling

Rolling helps to stimulate the balance organs in the inner ear. These are not well developed at birth, and movement activities help them to mature. Good balance is important for posture, control of muscles and coordination.

We're rolling all around	*Lie down on your back, lie baby on his*
Like a boat upon the sea,	*tummy on your abdomen with chest*
Roll, roll, roll,	*facing you, hold him in position with*
Roll, roll along with me.	*your arms. Roll from side to side, you*
(repeat)	*can roll more vigorously as the baby*
	develops stronger muscle tone!

Lift Me High and Swing Me Low   (GymbaROO)

This little action rhyme encourages moving the baby's body through space in different ways so he begins to learn about a range of spatial orientations. This is very stimulating for vision, balance, sound and touch.

Lift me high	*Standing up, hold baby up high*
And swing me low	*Swing baby between legs*
Round and round and round we go,	*Spin around with babe in arms*
Lift me high	
And swing me low	
Swinging fast and	*Swing baby from side to side –*
Swinging slow.	*fast and slow*

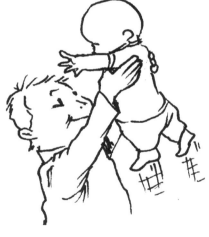

Wash the Dishes

Going upside down is loads of fun, and babies just love it (they were upside down in the womb for several months!). Start gently and get your baby used to a rolling movement first. It is a good idea to make sure your baby likes to go upside-down by holding him in your arms and leaning forward so baby's head tips back into the upside down position. Some babies may take a while to get used to the position. Just do a little upside-down movement every day to encourage familiarity with the position. Don't do upside-downs if your baby has a cold or is sick.

Wash the dishes,	*Lie baby on back, criss-cross the legs*
Dry the dishes	*Hold right leg crossed over the left*
Turn the dishes over.	*leg so the hip is encouraged to lift and baby will roll*
Wash the dishes	*Lie baby along your bent thighs as you sit on the floor, facing you*
Dry the dishes	*Lift legs one after the other*
Turn the dishes over.	*Lift baby upside down holding feet, bring back to rest on tummy across your legs*

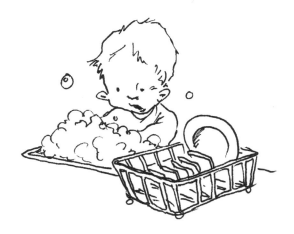

Hot Cross Buns

Hot cross buns!	*Hold baby's feet and criss-cross legs and feet over each other, then open out and cross the other way*
Hot-cross buns!	*Repeat*
One a penny, two a penny	*Stamp feet on the floor*
Hot-cross buns!	*Criss-cross legs and feet*
If ye have no daughters	*Criss-cross legs and feet*
Give them to your sons.	
One a penny, two a penny	*Clap feet together*
Hot-cross buns!	*Criss-cross legs and feet*

You can also do the criss-cross action with the hands and arms –
bring them across the chest.

Leg over Leg

This is a lovely little rhyme that helps babies feel what it is like to roll over from their back to their tummy.

Leg over leg as the dog went to Dover	*Lie baby on back, hold legs and cross over each other*
He came to a stile and – whoops –	*Cross one leg over the other and hold on the opposite side with foot touching the floor so the baby rolls over*
He went over!	

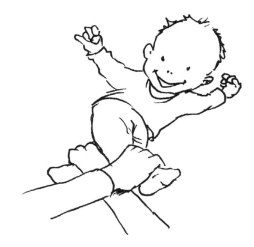

Father, Mother and Uncle Tom

Father, Mother and Uncle Tom	*Lie baby across legs*
Got on a pony and rode along	*Jiggle up and down*
Father fell off – whee	*Rock baby to one side*
Mother fell off – whee	*Rock baby to the other side*
But Uncle Tom went on and on and on and on and on …	*Jiggle up and down, and up and down until you or baby have had enough!*

Babies – mobile

Mobile babies, whether they are rolling, creeping or crawling, really begin to enjoy rhythm, music and action songs. They particularly enjoy the more vigorous movements, although both quieter and gentler sessions are important for them as well.

Massage

Once babies get themselves moving it is hard to stop them long enough to change their nappy let alone massage them! Try to keep the massage going, even if your little wriggler squirms away … you may just have to follow him around the room. Just after a bath or before bedtime often provide a marginally less wriggly opportunity! The trick is to keep the massage sessions short when your baby is restless and wants to get moving, and make the most of calmer times for longer sessions. Nappy change time is the perfect time for short and sweet little sessions!

Criss-Cross Apple Sauce

Touch is an important way for a baby to learn about his own body. This lovely rhyme is an absolute favourite! It really does give babies the goose bumps!

Criss-cross Apple Sauce	*Slide fingers across back from left shoulder to right hip, and right shoulder to left hip*
Spiders creeping down your back	*Creep fingers down back*
Cool breeze	*Open neck of shirt at the back and blow!*
Tight squeeze	*Give a hug from behind*
Giving you the shivers!	*Wriggle fingers all over back*

Weather

Rain is falling, rain is falling   *Tap child lightly with fingers on back*
Here it comes, here it comes
Pitter, pitter, patter
Pitter, pitter, patter
On your back, on your back.
Now it's pouring   *Firm tapping everywhere on child*
Now it's pouring
Plop, plop, plop   *Plop movements on body and head*
Plop, plop, plop
Now it's raining harder   *Plonk movements on arms and shoulders*
Now it's raining harder
Plonk, plonk, plonk
Plonk, plonk, plonk
Now there's lightning   *Zig-zag movements down the back*
Now there's lightning
Flash, flash, flash   *Whole palm: 'sizzling' movement down*
                               the legs

Flash, flash, flash
Then comes thunder   *Whole fist pressing* (Not too hard!
                               Watch for child's reaction)

Then comes thunder
Boom, boom, boom.

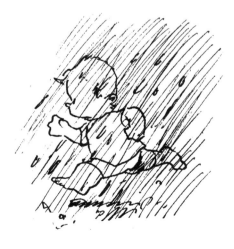

Knock at the Door

A nice short massage for the wriggling baby who wants to explore the world!

Knock at the door	*Tap lightly on the forehead*
Turn the lock	*Turn nose*
Wipe your feet	*Wipe finger under nose*
Open the door	*Open mouth*
Peek in!	*Look inside!*

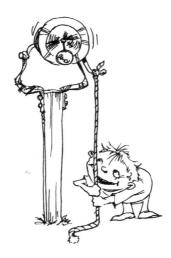

Spots

A leopard has got lots of spots,	*Make 'touch spots' all over baby's body*
What a lot of spots he's got	
A tiger has stripes, like long thin pipes	*Draw lines all over baby's body*
But a leopard has got lots of spots, spots, spots, spots.	*And back to spots*

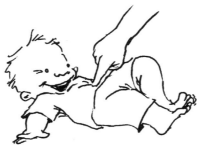

Shoe the Little Horse

This little poem has some hidden good advice for parents – our babies need to have bare feet for healthy foot development, so make sure that some time each day is spent without socks or shoes on!

Shoe the little horse　　　*Sit baby on your lap and pat the soles of*
the feet

Shoe the little mare
But let the little colt go
Bare, bare, bare.

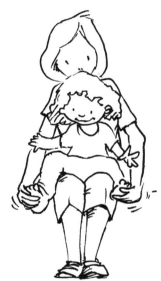

Action songs

Most children need assistance with moving many of their body parts in certain ways and in response to musical direction until they are over two years of age. You will find that, with lots of practice, our creeper-crawlers can learn to wave and clap!

Jack in the Box Jumps Up Like This

Jack in the box jumps up like this　　　　　　*Lift baby up high*
He makes me laugh when he waggles his head　*Tilt side to side*
Gently I push him down again　　　　　　　　*Tap gently on head*
But Jack in the box jumps up again!　　　　　　*Lift baby up again*

Giddy-up Horsey

Creeping and crawling babies just love to be moved, jiggled and bounced. This is an old favourite that babies love to repeat endlessly!

Giddy-up, giddy-up, giddy-up horsey

Sit with your knees bent up, baby sits on top, holding your hands

Giddy-up, giddy-up, Go! Go! Go!

Bounce your knees up and down

Giddy-up, giddy-up, giddy-up horsey
Giddy-up, giddy-up, Whoa! Whoa! Whoa!

Lean back, leaning baby forward

Jack and Jill

Jack and Jill went up the hill to fetch a pail of water

Sit baby on knees and gradually raise

Jack fell down and broke his crown

Open knees and baby plops onto the ground (support around waist)

And Jill came tumbling after.

Roll baby over and over

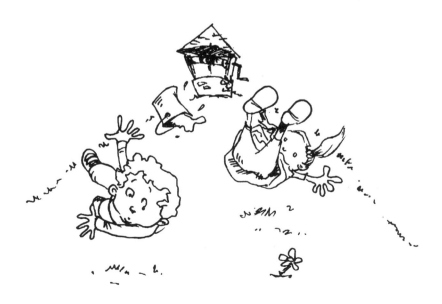

Jelly on the Plate

Jelly on the plate, jelly on the plate,

Wibble wobble, wibble wobble,
Jelly on the floor.

Sit baby on your bent knees as you sit on the floor
Wobble legs from side to side
Open legs, support baby under arms and baby gently plops onto the floor!

Biscuits in the tin, biscuits in the tin,
Shake shake, shake,
Shake shake, shake,
Biscuits in the tin.

Sit baby on bent knees
Shake knees up and down

Open knees and plop baby onto the floor

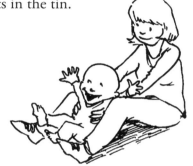

Tick-tock, Tick-tock, I'm a Little Cuckoo Clock

Rocking from side to side, and forward and backward on an unstable platform (a ball) helps develop balance. Movement and rhythm work together to stimulate the senses of hearing, sight, touch and balance.

Tick-tock, tick-tock,
I'm a little cuckoo
clock,

Child sitting on puff ball (a soft ball 30cm or larger). Hold around his waist

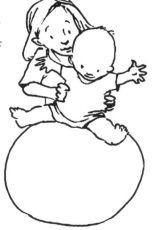

Tick-tock, tick-tock,
now it's one o'clock.
CUCKOO!
(Repeat, moving clock forward – two, three o'clock etc)
Lift twice for two
Lift three times for three

Rock child side to side

Lift up for CUCKOO

Ride a Cock Horse

Ride a cock horse to Banbury cross   *Lie baby across your legs and*
                                      gently bounce up and down
To see a fine lady upon a white horse,
With rings on her fingers and bells on her toes
She shall have music wherever she goes.

My hands are Clapping

My hands are clapping, clapping,   *Show your baby how to*
clapping,   *clap his hands*
My hands are clapping, just like this.
My feet are stamping, stamping,   *Stamp baby's feet on the*
stamping,   *floor*
My feet are stamping, just like this.
My arms are waving, waving, waving,   *Wave baby's arms in the air*
My arms are waving, just like this.
My legs are bending, bending, bending, *Bend baby's knees up and*
My legs are bending, just like this.   *down*

I Ride My Little Bicycle

I ride my little bicycle,   *Bicycle legs with baby lying on back*
I ride it to the shop,
And when I see a big red light   *(You can do this with arms as well)*
I know I have to stop!

Tap, Tap, Tap

Babies just love this one as they can bang on the table with their spoon! Little do they realize that the rhythmical tapping is training their brain for movement sequencing and memory development! Sit with your baby at the table, or across from him in his high chair. Start tapping on the surface as you sing:

Tap, tap, tapping on the table
Tap, tap, tapping on the table
Tap, tap, tapping on the table
Until it's time to stop!

On 'stop' raise your arms up. It won't be long before your baby does the same. For variety you can sometimes tap softly, or quite hard, fast or slowly. Baby will love imitating you, so you can do whatever your imagination suggests!

Hush-a-Bye Baby

Rhythm and beat are reinforced through movement. Rocking your baby from side to side, forwards and backwards and around and around helps your infant 'feel' the rhythm in action. He also hears you singing, and if you are holding him against your chest he will feel the rhythm through the vibrations of your body.

Hush-a-bye baby, on the tree top,	*Hold your baby up against your shoulder, rock your baby from side to side*
When the wind blows the cradle will rock;	
When the bough breaks the cradle will fall;	*Lower your baby down and up*
Down will come baby, bough, cradle and all.	
Rock-a-bye baby, thy cradle is green;	*Rock your baby forwards and backwards*
Father's a nobleman, Mother's a queen,	
Sister's a lady who wears a gold ring,	*Slowly spin with your baby, one way and then the other*
And Brother's a drummer who plays for the king.	
Hush-a-bye baby, way up on high;	*Lie baby tummy down along your arm – rock him from side to side*
Never mind baby, Mommy is nigh;	
Swinging the baby all around	*Slowly swing around on the spot, first one way and then the other*
Hush-a-bye baby, up hill and down.	*Raise baby up and down*

Toddlers

This age group just love to move. Most parents complain that they never seem to stop! The toddler years are the years of discovering how the body moves, refining balance and coordination and learning new skills. To do this the brain needs to repeatedly receive information about a particular action. Once the pattern of action is engrained in the brain then our toddlers can start to practise the next level of skill. As a result, they never seem to tire of the same action and embrace with their whole body anything that encourages them to move!

If You're Happy and You Know It

This is a very old song that still enthrals children. Just follow the lyrics and you will know what to do!

If you're happy and you know it clap your hands
If you're happy and you know it clap your hands
If you're happy and you know it and you really want to show it
If you're happy and you know it clap your hands.

Additional verses
Stamp your feet; wave your arms; tap your toes; turn around; do a somersault!

Grandfather Clock   (GymbaROO)

Rhythm and timing are important for the internal body clock to regulate itself and for developing the capacity to time movements smoothly. This is called 'temporal awareness'. Temporal awareness is important for many areas of development, including understanding concepts such as up/down, in/out and left/right – all essential for later learning skills such as reading, writing and maths concepts.

The Grandfather clock goes tick … tock … tick … tock …	*Say slowly, children have arms out and tick-tock from side to side*
The kitchen clock goes tick tock, tick tock, tick tock, tick tock	*Say more quickly, children jump up and down on the spot*
All the little watches go tick, tick, tick, tick, tick, tick, tick.	*Say very fast as children jump in circles.*

Roly Poly

Roly poly, roly poly, ever so slowly. *Roll hands slowly over each other*
Roly poly, roly poly faster, faster,   *Roll hands quickly*
faster and ...
STOP!   *Stop and clap*

Turn Around

(to the tune of Frère Jacques)

Turn around, turn around
Touch your toes, touch your toes
Do a little jumping, Do a little jumping
Then bob down, then bob down.

There Were Ten in the Bed

There were ten in the bed,   *Hold up ten fingers*
And the little one said:
'Roll over! Roll over!'   *Roll arms over and over, or roll
                                   whole body over*

So they all rolled over,
And one fell out.   *Hold up one finger*

There were nine, eight, seven, six, five, four, three, two, one ...

There were none in the bed,
So no one said:
'Roll over! Roll over!'

I Hear Thunder (tune of 'Where is Thumbkin')

I hear thunder, I hear thunder,   *Firmly pat hands on back*
Hark don't you, hark don't you?   *Put hand to ear as if listening*
Pitter patter raindrops,   *Lightly tap back with pitter patter
                                   of fingers*

Pitter patter raindrops,
I'm wet through,   *Hug self*
So are you!   *Hug toddler*

The Ants Go Marching

Marching around the room is not only great for development, but the little ones love it! Most will not really 'march' at this age, since this movement is not patterned into the brain until between the age of 3 and 5 ... but this does not stop little ones from having a great time!

The ants go marching one by one, Hoorah! Hoorah!	*'March' around the room*
The ants go marching one by one, Hoorah! Hoorah!	
The ants go marching one by one,	
The little one stops to suck his thumb,	*Pretend to suck thumb*
And they all go marching down into the ground	
To get out of the rain.	
Boom, boom, boom, boom!	*Stamp feet on the ground*

Additional verses

The ants go marching two by two	
... the little one stopped to tie his shoe	*Bend down to touch toes*
The ants go marching three by three	
... the little stopped to climb a tree.	*Lift legs up alternatively*

Moving

Fishes swim in water clear,	*Extend arms out front, join hands and waggle*
Birds fly in the air,	*Flap arms up and down*
Serpents creep along the ground,	*Lie on tummy and wriggle on floor*
While children run around and around	*Jump up and go for a run!*

Horsey, Horsey

Our little ones are not yet galloping, but they will try their best to run as fast as they can without falling over. Try not to hold onto your child's hand. This throws his balance off to one side, making it hard for him to develop good balancing skills.

Horsey, horsey, don't you stop,	*Gallop around the room*
Just let your feet go clippety clop;	
Your tail goes swish,	
As we gallop along.	
Giddy-up, you're homeward bound!	

Jack, Be Nimble

Using this traditional rhyme enables us to encourage older toddlers (age two to two-and-a-half) to do a movement activity other than just run. It is actually quite challenging for them to stop and engage in another movement. Get them to 'stop' before attempting to leap.

Jack, be nimble,	*Run around the room*
Jack, be quick,	
Jack jump over	*Pretend to leap over an object*
The candlestick.	

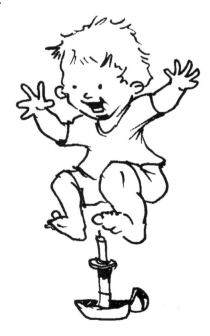

Row, Row, Row Your Boat

This is a great rhyme for helping develop upper body strength. Strong neck, shoulders and arms are important for strong hands and fingers. This is important for pencil grip, pencil control, handwriting and drawing. Start from the seated position. Once your child is strong enough you can do this standing up. To help prevent feet from slipping, your child can stand on your feet!

Row, row, row your boat,	*Sit opposite your child, knees bent, feet touch and holding hands*
Gently down the stream.	*Rock backwards and forwards*
Merrily, merrily, merrily, merrily,	
Life is but a dream.	
Row, row, row your boat,	*Rock backward and forward as above*
Gently down the stream.	
If you see a crocodile	
Don't forget to scream!	*All scream !*
Row, row, row your boat,	*Rock backwards and forwards as above*
Gently down the stream.	
Ha, ha, tricked you!	
It's a submarine!	

Ring-a-Ring-a-Roses

This much-loved nursery rhyme is so popular with the toddlers that I think we could do it for a whole 45-minute class! It's a great way of learning to time movement. Initially many of the toddlers will fall down or jump up too soon ... but they quickly learn to wait for the right moment! Timing movement is important for many thinking skills and motor coordination.

Ring-a-ring-a-roses,	*Hold hands and move around in a circle*
Pocket full of posies,	
Atishoo! Atishoo!	
We all fall down!	*Fall down*
The cows are in the meadow	*Lie on the ground*
Eating buttercups	
Atishoo! Atishoo!	
We all jump up!	*Jump up!*

Preschoolers

Preschoolers are refining the movements they have already learned as their brains prepare for more sophisticated levels of learning. Rhythm and movement play a very important role in the development of this age group as the brain responds far more to song than it does to speech, and movement accompanying rhyme or song provides additional stimulus to the information the brain receives and stores.

Clap Your Hands – Touch Your Toes

Following the actions in the rhyme is great for developing a preschooler's listening skills and ability to smoothly follow one action after another. If they repeat an action rhyme regularly they will begin to anticipate the next action without even thinking about it!

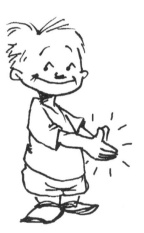

Clap your hands,
Touch your toes,
Turn around
And put your finger on your nose.
Flap your arms,
Jump up high,
Wiggle your fingers
And reach for the sky!

Let Everyone Clap Hands Like Me

Preschoolers love having the chance to make up the action that everyone is to copy, so let them! This little rhyme aids in the development of visualization and helps children to develop an internal body awareness of timing and rhythm.

Let everyone clap hands like me,
It's easy as easy can be.
Come on and join in with the game,
You'll find that it's always the same.

You can make up many more verses:

Let everyone

stand up like me
spin around like me
jump up like me
pull faces like me
hop hopping like me

The Wheels on the Bus

An enormously popular song with all age groups, it is not until they reach age three that children can independently carry out all the actions to this fun song. Crying like a baby seems to be particularly amusing to this age group!

The wheels on the bus go round and round, Round and round, round and round. The wheels on the bus go round and round All the way to town.	*Roll hands and arms over and over*

Additional verses

The people on the bus stand up, sit down	*Children stand up, sit down*
The wipers on the bus go swish, swish, swish	*Use arms to swish from side to side*
The babies on the bus go 'wah, wah, wah'	*Squish up face* and *cry out 'wah, wah, wah'*
The horn on the bus goes beep, beep, beep.	*Push hand and palm away from body*

Forward Roll Rhyme

Forward somersaults are a fun way of stimulating the balance mechanisms in the inner ear and assist with the maturation of posture. This little rhyme assists our preschoolers to time their movements so that the forward roll is performed smoothly and carefully.

I can stand on one leg.	*Stand on one leg*
I can stand on two,	*Stand with two legs apart*
I can bend over,	*Bend over, hands on the floor*
And look right through.	*Look through legs and gently roll onto back*

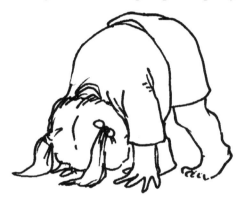

Teddy Bear (version 1)

Turning around on the spot is another way of helping the body learn how to balance – and this age group just love spinning!

Teddy bear, teddy bear, turn around.	*Turn on the spot*
Teddy bear, teddy bear, touch the ground.	*Bend down and touch the ground*
Teddy bear, teddy bear reach up high.	*Reach up high with hands, stand on tip-toe*
Teddy bear, teddy bear, touch the sky.	*Wave hands in the air*

Turn Around and Touch the Ground

Another fun spinning rhyme!

Turn around and touch the ground,
Turn around and touch the ground,
Turn around and touch the ground,
And fall right down!

Teddy Bear (version 2)

Teddy bear, teddy bear turn around,	*Turn around on the spot*
Teddy bear, teddy bear, touch the ground,	*Bend over and touch the floor*
Teddy bear teddy bear touch your nose,	*Touch nose*
Teddy bear, teddy bear, touch your toes,	*Touch toes*
Teddy bear, teddy bear climb the stairs,	*Pretend to climb the stairs*
Teddy bear, teddy bear, say your prayers,	*Hands together in prayer position*
Teddy bear, teddy bear, turn out the light,	*Pull one hand and arm in downward motion*
Teddy bear, teddy bear, say goodnight!	*Blow a kiss!*

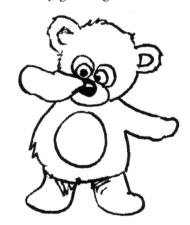

Rocking and Rolling

I'm rocking all around like a boat on the sea,	*Child lies on back, legs drawn up to chest, arms holding legs*
Rock, rock, rock, rock, rock along with me.	*Rock to and fro for remainder of song*
I'm rocking all around like a boat on the sea.	
Rocking, rocking, rocking, rocking, rock.	

or

I'm rolling all around like a boat on the sea,
Roll, roll, roll, roll, roll along with me.
I'm rolling all around like a boat on the sea,
Rolling, rolling, rolling, rolling, rolling, roll.

Child lies in log or pencil roll position, arms up above head, body and legs straight, then roll over and over. Roll back in the opposite direction for the second half of the song. This helps to reduce dizziness and stimulates the balance organs in the inner ear.

An Elephant

Preschoolers just love imitating animals, and this action rhyme can be modified to include any animals that you – or they – can think of!

An elephant goes like this and that.	*On all fours moving around slowly*
He's terribly big,	*Stand, reach up tall*
And he's terribly fat.	*Reach hands out wide*
He has no fingers,	*Fist hands, hiding fingers*
He has no toes,	*Wiggle toes*
But goodness, gracious, what a nose!	*Nose to arm and swing as if a trunk*

Finger plays and action rhymes

All children love finger plays and action rhymes – from the smallest of babies to the school-age child. There's just something about them that children really enjoy – even if they do get their fingers tied in a knot! But finger plays, foot plays and action rhymes are more than just fun, they help in the development of early speech, rhythm and timing, dramatization skills, co-ordination of hand or foot movement and body awareness. Finger plays also help to develop hand and finger strength and coordination, necessary for correctly holding and controlling a pencil when drawing and writing at school. Finger plays and action rhymes are also a great way to encourage communication between an adult and a child, and can be very effective in helping shy children participate in a group situation, as they concentrate on their own body and its actions.

Rhymes also provide the basis for the development of good listening skills. The words and actions of rhymes are introduced simultaneously so that the words are supported by the action, and children derive a great deal of pleasure from coordinating hand/foot or body movements with the rhythm of the verse.

When playing finger and foot rhymes with children, it is important to realize that children will be aware of their hands and feet before they are aware of their fingers and toes. This means that the young child will not be able to manipulate his fingers and toes until he has learnt where his hands and feet are. Only after a child knows where his body parts are can he begin to move them individually.

If your child is having difficulty with finger plays, remember that the fingers are an extension of the hand, arm, shoulder and back muscles and if these are not well developed, finger control will be much more difficult. Try to engage in activities that strengthen the muscles in the back, shoulder and arm, and this will help your child develop strength and control in his fingers.

Individual movement of the toes is not as easy as movement of the fingers, so the aim is to get the toes wriggling freely and easily independently of foot movement. Foot and toe movement is dependent on the flexibility of the larger muscles of the hips, legs and ankles.

Finger puppets make the activity even more fun, and help children focus on the finger that needs to be moved. If you don't have any finger puppets at home, you can draw a face on your child's finger – or cut off the fingers from a rubber glove and draw on a face. Hand puppets are fabulous for full hand-movement action rhymes – all you need is an old sock and a thick pen to draw on eyes, nose and mouth. Or, if you are feeling more adventurous, sew on cloth features and some wool for hair!

Finger rhymes for babies

Babies love hand and finger rhymes – with parents actively doing the movements with and on their child, tickling their skin and wriggling their fingers and toes. Two action rhymes seem to be deeply embedded in the English cultural history: 'This Little Piggy Went to Market', and 'Round and Round the Garden' (see p. 83) – but there are many other wonderful rhymes too that babies love.

This Little Piggy Went to Market

This little piggy went to market,	*Waggle your baby's big toe*
This little piggy stayed at home,	*Waggle second toe*
This little piggy ate roast beef,	*Waggle third toe*
While this little piggy had none.	*Waggle fourth toe*
And this little piggy went	*Waggle little toe*
Whee, whee, whee, all the way home.	*Tickle baby up their body to under their arms*

Or try this less traditional version:

This little pig had a rub-a-dub-dub,	*Rub big toe*
This little pig had a scrub-a-scrub-scrub,	*Rub second toe*
This little pig called out 'Bears!'	*Gently pull third toe*
Down came the jar with a loud slam-bang,	*Clap whole foot between hands*
And this little pig had all the jam!	*Wiggle little toe*

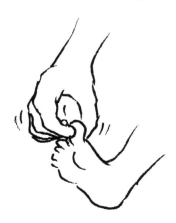

Ten Little Fingers

I have ten little fingers and ten little toes,   *Touch each body part as*
                                                   you say the rhyme

Two little arms and one little nose,
One little mouth and two little ears,
Two little eyes for smiles and tears,
One little head and two little feet,
One little chin makes me all complete!

Fe Fi Fo Fum

Finger awareness follows awareness of arms. Toe awareness follows
awareness of legs.
Fe fi fo fum, now I've got you by the   *Hold and wriggle baby's*
thumb.   *thumbs*
Eeney Meeney Miney Moe,
Now I've got you by the toe   *Hold and wriggle toes!*

One, two, three, four five

One, two, three, four, five,   *Wiggle each of baby's finger in turn as*
                                you count

Once I caught a fish alive;
Six, seven eight nine, ten,
Then I let him go again.
Why did you let him go?   *Stroke baby's hand*
Because he bit my finger so.   *Make nibbling motions on baby's hand*
                                or fingers

Which finger did he bite?
This little finger on my   *Wiggle baby's little finger*
right.   *on the right hand*

My Hands are Clapping

My hands are clapping, clapping, clapping;
My hands are clapping, just like this.

My feet are stamping, stamping, stamping;
My feet are stamping, just like this

My arms are waving, waving, waving;
My arms are waving, just like this.

You can help your baby to do all of these movements. Remember these larger body movements develop before the finer movements of the fingers and hands, so this is a great starting point for finger games and action rhymes.

Finger rhymes for toddlers

Children first need to do songs and rhymes which involve the movement of the hands and feet as a whole – such as clapping hands together, shaking hands, rolling hands around each other and using them to tap on other large body parts like their knees, or tummy – before they can progress to finger rhymes.

Twinkle, Twinkle, Little Star   (Jane Taylor)

A favourite for many years, *Twinkle, Twinkle Little Star* is the perfect finger rhyme for toddlers. They can manipulate their hands as whole and act out the full body moves as they reach up high. Some of the younger toddlers will have difficulty with forming the star, but lots of practice and maturity means they will soon learn!

Twinkle, twinkle little star,   *Twinkle fingers above head*
How I wonder what you are.
Up above the world so high,   *Point up to the sky*
Like a diamond in the sky.   *Make a star shape between two*
    thumbs and two pointer fingers

Twinkle, twinkle, little star,   *Twinkle fingers above head*
How I wonder what you are.

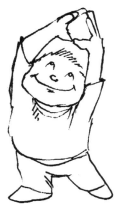

Learning to individually manipulate each finger is quite a challenge for our toddlers. They learn control of their thumb and pointer (index) fingers first, then little finger, and finally 'tall man' and 'ring man' (definitely the hardest!) As stated, children need excellent fine motor control of their fingers to hold their pencil correctly, grip it with the right amount of tension and to carefully manipulate other objects, such as a ruler, pencil sharpener or scissors.

You can then introduce movement of the thumb with the hands, such as 'Where is thumbkin?' where the child 'hides' his thumb in the middle of his fingers and then holds it upright for all to see. Don't expect movement of the other fingers just yet – that takes quite a bit of developmental skill that usually doesn't occur until after the child is two-and-a-half to three. From that age you can begin to introduce 'tall man' and 'ring man', and during age three, games using individual fingers should be possible, even if cautiously at first.

Where is Thumbkin?

Where is thumbkin, where is thumbkin?	*Hold hands behind back. Help child to get thumb ready in position, remainder of fingers are curled into a fist*
Here I am, here I am!	*Bring out right and then left hand with thumbs pointing up*
How are you this morning? Very well, I thank you.	*Bend right thumb up and down towards left thumb and then bend left thumb up and down towards right thumb*
Run away, run away.	*Return right hand to behind back, then left hand*
Where is Pointer, where is Pointer?	*As above, this time have the pointer fingers ready, thumb tucked in with other fingers*

Here I am, here I am!
How are you this morning? Very well, I thank you.
Run away, run away.

Tommy Thumb

Tommy Thumb,	*Hand forms a fist*
Tommy Thumb,	
Where are you?	
Here I am, here I am,	*Thumb held out*
How do you do?	*Bend thumb up and down*

Tommy Thumbs

Tommy thumbs up, tommy thumbs down,	*Thumbs up, thumbs down*
Tommy thumbs dancing all around the town.	*Wiggling thumbs*
Dancing on your shoulder,	*Dance thumbs on shoulder*
Dancing on your head,	*Dance thumbs on head*
Dancing on your knees	*Dance thumbs on knees*
Now, tuck them into bed.	*Tuck thumbs under arms*

Incy Wincy Spider

Toddlers can be encouraged to move their own hands and arms. Preschoolers may be able to move their fingers up each other like a web. Parents can move their own fingers and arms, creeping them up the baby's trunk, arms or legs.

Incy wincy spider	*Climb fingers up body*
Climbed up the waterspout.	
Down came the rain	*Wiggle fingers in the air from high to low*
and washed the spider out!	
Out came the sun shine	*Over head, arms up and open out wide*
and dried up all the rain.	*Arms down low and then up high*
So incy wincy spider	
Climbed up the spout again.	*Walk fingers up body*

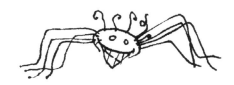

The Finger Family

Peter Pointer	*Child attempts to hold up each finger as it is called out loud*
Toby Tall	
Ruby Ring	
Baby Finger	
Finger Family – here we are.	

Grandma's Glasses

Here are grandma's glasses,	*Make circles with thumb and pointer finger and hold up to eyes*
Here is grandma's hat.	*Hold hand together on top of head*
This is how she folds her hands	*Fold arms*
And lays them in her lap.	*Lay hands in lap*

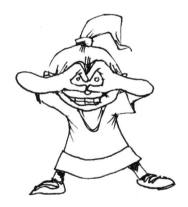

Reach Up

Reach up to the sky,	*Reach up tall*
Reach down to the ground.	*Touch hands to the floor*
Hold out your arms and	*Hold arms out straight to the sides*
Turn round and round.	*Spin slowly around and around*

Finger rhymes for preschoolers

By the time a child is four, finger games come into their own. This age group have much better control of each individual finger and can manipulate them accordingly, so finger games and rhymes – while still challenging – can be managed without adult assistance. With practice, most can competently manage a range of simple finger plays and action rhymes. To enhance the enjoyment further, children love the addition of finger puppets!

Two Fat Gentlemen

Being able to control fingers independently is an essential component of fine motor coordination. Our three- and four-year-olds love finger rhymes and songs as they are beginning to be able to control each of their fingers ... although 'tall man' and 'ring finger' are a bit tricky still!

Two fat gentlemen met in a lane,	*Hold both hands up to face each other*
Bowed most politely, bowed once again.	*Thumbs bow towards each other*
How do you do?	
How do you do?	
How do you do again?	

Additional verses

Two thin ladies	*Pointers*
Two little school boys	*Little finger*

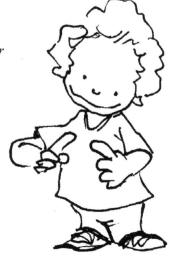

One, Two, Three, Four, Five

One, two, three, four, five, *Hold up one finger at a time – or carer can touch each finger*

Once I caught a fish alive.
Six, seven, eight, nine, ten, *Hold up each finger of the other hand*
Then I let it go again.
Why did you let it go?
Because it bit my finger so! *Shake hand up and down*
Which finger did it bite?
This little finger on the right! *Hold out 'pinkie' finger*

Johnny Works With One Hammer

This little rhyme gets more difficult with every verse, so is a good one for the progression of skills. The older the toddler, the more verses you can include. Start with just one fist and then two fists hammering.

Johnny works with one hammer, one, hammer, one hammer.
Johnny works with one hammer, then he works with two.

Johnny works with two hammers, two hammers, two hammers.
Johnny works with two hammers, then he works with three.

etc

Last verse:

Johnny works with five hammers … then he goes to sleep.

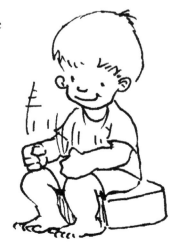

Sing this sitting down. The actions are as follows:
One hammer – pound one fist on knee
Two hammers – pound two fists on knees
Three hammers – two fists, one foot
Four hammers – two fists, two feet
Five hammers – two fists, two feet, nod head
Then he goes to sleep – hands form pillow on which to lay head

Miss Polly Had a Dolly

Preschoolers adore this action rhyme!

Miss Polly had a dolly who was sick, sick, sick,	*Fold arms and rock pretend dolly*
So she called for the doctor to come quick, quick, quick.	*One hand to ear and one 'dialling' the telephone*
The doctor came with his bag and his hat,	*One hand swings bag, the other holds hat on*
And he knocked on the door with a rat-a-tat-tat.	*Knock one fist on palm of other hand*
He looked at the dolly and he shook his head,	*Shake head back and forward*
He said, 'Miss Polly put her straight to bed'.	*Shake finger up and down*
He wrote on his paper for a pill, pill, pill,	*Write with finger on palm of other hand*
That will make her better, yes it will, will, will.	*Nod vigorously*

Little Peter Rabbit

Little Peter Rabbit	*Waggle both hands on the top of the head like floppy rabbit ears*
Has a fly upon his nose,	*Touch nose*
Little Peter Rabbit	*Repeat above*
Has a fly upon his nose,	
Little Peter Rabbit	*Repeat*
Has a fly upon his nose,	
And he flicked it and he flopped it and it flew away.	*Flop hand from side to side in front of face*

Two Little Dickey Birds

This is a favourite of preschoolers. Something about these little birds being called 'Peter' and 'Paul' seems to tickle their fancy! They are also learning to remember right from left and which hand is 'Peter' and which hand is 'Paul'. Memory sequencing is important for learning maths and for understanding stories.

Two little dickey birds	*Have hands closed, pointer finger out,*
sitting on a wall,	*resting against shoulders or knees*
One called Peter	*Waggle the finger of the right hand*
One called Paul.	*Waggle the finger of the left hand*
Fly away Peter.	*Waggle right finger as moved behind back*
Fly away Paul.	*Waggle left finger as moved behind back*
Come back Peter.	*Bring right hand back to shoulder or knee*
Come back Paul.	*Bring left hand back to shoulder or knee*

Where is Thumbkin?

Building skills through 'layered learning', we can use rhymes such as this one, which we had earlier, and develop further skills. The first two verses can be managed by toddlers, but it is not until the children gain fine motor control in all their fingers that they can manage the tall finger, ring finger and little finger.

Where is Thumbkin, where is Thumbkin?	*Hold hands behind back. Help child to get thumb ready in position, remainder of fingers are curled into a fist*
Here I am, here I am!	*Bring out right and then left hand with thumbs pointing up*
How are you this morning?	*Bend right thumb up and down towards left thumb and then bend left*
Very well, I thank you.	*left thumb up and down towards right thumb*
Run away, run away.	*Return right hand to behind back, then left hand*
Where is Pointer, where is Pointer?	*As above, this time have the pointer fingers ready, thumb tucked in with other fingers*

Here I am, here I am!
How are you this morning? Very well, I thank you.
Run away, run away.

Where is Tall Man, where is Tall Man?
Here I am, here I am!
How are you this morning? Very well, I thank you.
Run away, run away.

Where is Ring Man, where is Ring Man?
Here I am, here I am!
How are you this morning? Very well, I thank you.
Run away, run away.

Where is Pinkie, where is Pinkie?
Here I am, here I am!
How are you this morning? Very well, I thank you.
Run away, run away.

Where is the family, where is the family?
Here we are, here we are!
How are you this morning? Very well, we thank you.
Run away, run away.

One Finger and Thumb Keep Moving

This action song is quite challenging as it asks our preschooler to move more and more body parts at the same time!

One finger and thumb keep moving.   *Move one finger and one thumb*
One finger and thumb keep moving.
One finger and thumb keep moving.
And we'll all be merry and bright.
Two fingers, two thumbs keep   *now move two fingers and two*
moving etc.   *thumbs together*

(Repeat as above)
Two arms, two fingers, two thumbs, etc.
Two legs, two arms, two fingers, two thumbs, etc.
One head, two legs, two arms, two fingers, two thumbs, etc.

Ten Little Monkeys

This is a firm favourite of preschoolers. There are ten verses and they never get bored! Be prepared because you will have to do this one over and over again!

Ten little monkeys jumping on   *Hold ten fingers up, bounce hands*
the bed,   *up and down*

One fell off and bumped his head!	*Tap forehead with heel of one hand*
Mama called the doctor and the doctor said	*Use finger as if pushing buttons on the phone*
'No more monkeys, Jumping on the bed!'	*Pointer (index) finger out and hand movement up and down as if being told off!*

Nine little monkeys jumping on the bed etc
Eight … Seven … Six … Five … Four … Three … Two … One …
No more monkeys jumping on the bed!

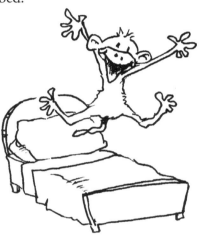

Five Little Fishes

Five little fishes swimming in pool;	*Hold up five fingers*
The first one said, 'This pool is cool'.	*Wiggle thumb, fold down*
The second one said, 'This pool is deep'.	*Wiggle pointer finger, fold down*
The third one said 'I want to sleep'.	*Fold tall finger down*
The fourth one said, 'Let's take a dip'.	*Fold ring finger down*
The fifth one said, 'I spy a ship'.	*5 fingers up. Look through hands like spyglass*
Fisherboat comes,	*Cup hands together and wave along like a boat on the sea*
Line goes ker-splash	*Pretend to throw fishing line*
Away the five little fishes dash.	*Wiggle five fingers away*

CHAPTER 5

Poetry and Fairy Stories

Before the invention of the printing press, books were rare, valuable and treasured items, and only a relatively small percentage of the population was able to read and write. Knowledge, history, religious beliefs, cultural traditions, wisdom and folklore were largely handed down to the next generation through the medium of oral language. In earlier chapters we have already seen how much of this was done through song, poetry, ballads, pictures and, of course, the telling of stories.

As the digital age encourages increasing dependence on visual images as a primary information medium, it is easy to forget that visual information is processed differently from auditory information. One of the features of visual information processing is that it tends to be rapid and capable of absorbing large amounts of information quickly; but it can also be quickly erased when new information comes in, partly to prevent information overload.

Information received through the auditory channel tends to be processed more slowly but to go in more deeply. This is illustrated when typing something at speed onto a computer screen. When checking for errors on the screen, the brain often 'sees' what it thinks it should have typed, and it is easy to miss mistakes. If, on the other hand, you read the text aloud, the speed of processing is slower, more accurate in picking up details, and typing errors are detected. Similarly, it is often easier to remember the *details* of a story that has been read aloud, whereas in remembering a film you are more likely to recall the *gist* or specific *scenes*.

When information is absorbed through the aural channel, in order to 'make sense' of the sounds they must be translated into visual images in the mind's eye. This process of forming mental pictures attaches new information to something already known, a way of embedding new information into old, something I referred to previously as 'layered learning'. It also involves both hemispheres of the brain. Matching auditory to visual mental images, and visual to auditory, is essential to processes of reading and writing. Listening also requires focused attention (receptive stillness). Those of us who are old enough to remember the regular afternoon radio programme 'Listen with Mother' will remember that the story part always began with: 'Are you sitting comfortably? Then I'll begin.'

In earlier chapters we saw how both the mother's and father's voice are important acoustic links between pre- and post-natal life, and how the music of the voice implies meaning and conveys emotions far beyond the child's understanding of vocabulary. In this way, stories and poems which use long words help introduce children to complex, nuanced language.

But there is far more to the telling of stories than the development of brain mechanisms. Stories admit children to a particular culture, set of values, and vernacular. Stereotypes of good and evil, rich and poor, vanity and valour, pride and greed help children to understand the strengths and weaknesses inherent in human nature. Children naturally tend to side with the 'goody' and enjoy the anticipation and struggle that takes place between 'once upon a time' and 'they all lived happily ever after'. But besides this 'moral' aspect of stories, old fairytales often speak intuitively and imaginatively to the child's experience, developmental stages, fears and concerns. They are also invariably patterned in a particular, rhythmic, repetitive and even ritualized way, for instance as embodied in the 'three sons' who each set out on a journey, or the 'good' and 'bad' daughter who meet the same sequence of trials and respond to them differently. Such repetition nurtures both security and expectancy in a child, giving her a sense of pattern, order and meaning in which she can participate.

When I was teaching adults in Germany a number of years ago I asked a member of the group whether traditional fairy stories were being abandoned because they were thought too scary for children, or out of fear of demonizing minority groups. He was shocked at the suggestion, saying that in Germany fairy stories were a treasured part of childhood, *one* of whose benefits being that, through imaginative empathy, they taught children the difference between right and wrong, and nurtured moral behaviour. These are the hallmarks of a civilized society.

Fairy tales appeal directly to the imagination, invoking imaginative archetypes that may only indirectly find their way into our moral actions. 'Moral fables' on the other hand directly aim at what we may regard as a more superficial kind of moral instruction, through warning of possible consequences, and as such are more suited to somewhat older children. Such 'cautionary tales' thus provide more direct commentary on behaviour. *Struwwelpeter* ('Shock-headed Peter') provides one example of this; it was written by Heinrich Hoffmann, a German psychiatrist. In 1844 Hoffman had wanted to buy a picture book for his son for Christmas. Unimpressed by what he saw, he purchased a notebook and wrote his own stories with pictures instead. Each story has a clear moral, which demonstrates the extreme consequences of misbehaviour.

As a small child who was addicted to sucking my fingers at the time, the picture of Struwwelpeter on the front cover of the book with his thumbs cut off *did* frighten me, but the other stories made me aware of the dangers of silly behaviour without fear and without the need for a health and safety policy to cover every eventuality. While parents are often alarmed at these tales, children are generally enthralled by them, and rather than taking them too literally can generalize their wider relevance.

The Story of Fidgety Philip
from Heinrich Hoffman's Struwwelpeter[1]

Let me see if Philip can
Be a little gentleman;
Let me see, if he is able
To sit still for once at table:
Thus papa bade Philip behave;
And Mamma looked very grave.
But fidgety Phil,
He won't sit still:
He wriggles
And giggles,

And then I declare,
Swings backwards and forwards
And tilts his chair,
Just like any rocking horse:
'Philip! I am getting cross!'

See the naughty, restless child
Growing still more rude and wild.
Till his chair falls over quite.
Philip screams with all his might.
Catches at the cloth, but then
That makes matters worse again.
Down upon the ground they fall.
Glasses, plates, knives, forks and all.
How Mama did fret and frown.
When she saw them tumbling down!
And Papa made such a face!
Philip is in sad disgrace.

Where is Philip, where is he?
Fairly cover'd up you see!
Cloth and all are lying on him;
What a terrible to-do!
Dishes, glasses, snapt in two!
Here a knife and there a fork!
Philip, this is cruel work.
Table all so bare, and ah!
Poor Papa, and poor Mama
Look quite cross, and wonder how
They shall make their dinner now.

Each of the stories focuses on an aspect of child behaviour that has vexed adults for generations: thumb-sucking, fidgeting, fussy eating, inattention, and playing with fire. While the language appeals to adult humour, the exaggerated features of the behaviour and the reaction of adults in the stories appeals to children. Even quite young children are able to recognize the element of wilful disobedience in Fidgety Phil's behaviour. While there can be many other reasons for fidgeting, thumbsucking and inattention which can be resolved by understanding the underlying causes, the moral of *this* tale is the child's disregard for the needs of others. One hundred and sixty years after it was written, this child might receive a diagnosis of Attention Deficit Hyperactivity Disorder (ADHD), whereas the stories acknowledge that some obnoxious behaviour is a normal part of children's development, and that teaching old-fashioned values such as consideration for others still has an important place in children's upbringing.

Why bedtime stories matter

The tradition of reading a bedtime story is in decline in the United Kingdom. A survey carried out for Granada TV in the north-west of England in 2006 revealed that, by their own admission, forty per cent of parents never read to their child. I see this increasingly when discussing children's reading problems with parents. Part of the remedial developmental movement programme we offer them often involves reading their child a bedtime story every night. One family, stunned by the suggestion, remarked, 'But that means I will have to read to *all* my children. We have never done that.'

Rachel Williams in *The Guardian* in April 2010 reported that:

> More than half of primary teachers say they have seen at least one child with no experience of being told stories at home [...] One literacy expert branded the findings a 'national disaster', warning that such children were at risk of being left behind at school and failing to develop the creative talents needed to lead happy and productive lives. Pie Corbett, who acts as an educational adviser to the government, said too many children were left to watch TV instead of being read a bedtime story, often by busy middle-class parents. Corbett said: 'This isn't just an economic thing – it's not just people who come from poor backgrounds, it's across the whole of society. You get a lot of children coming from very privileged backgrounds who've spent a lot of time in front of the TV and not enough time snuggled up with a good book. The TV does the imagining for you – and it doesn't care whether you're

listening or not.' Research shows that children who are read to on a regular basis before they start school are most likely to succeed. 'It's a key predictor in terms of educational success,' said Corbett. Being told stories boosts language and, by feeding the child's imagination, develops abstract thought. 'Children who are told stories are the ones who first form abstract concepts across the curriculum – in other words, being read to makes you brainy,' Corbett said. 'The best writers in the class are always those who are avid readers.' He said parents needed to get the message that reading really matters. 'It may be parents have lost faith with this idea, but education is a way out of poverty.' Reading levels have improved in recent years, but attainment in writing has not kept up. Nearly two-thirds of the 300 teachers questioned by Oxford University Press said children were less able to tell stories in writing than ten years ago. One teacher responding to the survey said: 'Where are all the parents who sing and recite nursery rhymes to their children? We have created a generation who are failing to give their children the phonological start they need to become a capable reader.' Another said: 'There are children who have had very few stories read to them and I notice that now many do not know the traditional fairy tales – beyond Walt Disney cartoons that is.'[2]

Simple stories told over and over again help children establish a bedtime routine and wind down at the end of the day, and create space for parent and child to spend a few treasured minutes together every day sharing an activity and language which goes beyond more mundane, daily conversation. Some of the best bedtime stories, that have stood the test of time, tend to draw on musical language, imagination and repetition. The American children's book *Goodnight Moon*[3] by Margaret Wise Brown is a good example of the genre, and is a much-loved favourite with children.

Extract from *Goodnight Moon* by Margaret Wise Brown

In the great green room
There was a telephone
And a red balloon

And a picture of –
The cow jumping over the moon
And there were three little bears sitting on chairs
And a comb and a brush, a bowl of mush
And a quiet old lady who was whispering 'hush'
Goodnight room.

The story continues by saying 'good night' to all the familiar objects in the room: the light, the red balloon, the clocks, the socks, the brush, the comb, the stars, the air and 'the noises everywhere'. This story becomes a part of bedtime routine, the ritual of saying good night to all the familiar things is a calming process in the drift towards sleep. The child also plays an active role, remembering the rhyme, the objects and the sequence, while repetition of rhyming words improves auditory discrimination and vocabulary.

Other stories help to develop children's observation and creative imagination. In *A Little House of Your Own*,[4] Beatrice Schenk de Regners introduces children to the idea that:

Everyone has to have a little house of his own.
Every boy has to have his own little house.
Every girl should have a little house
All to herself …
There are many kinds of
secret houses. There are
many places where you can have your own little house.
This is what I mean …
Behind a chair in a corner
can be a good house.
A big hat is like
A little house …
Your papa is in *his*
Own little house when
He is behind his newspaper.
He wants everyone to leave him
alone. He doesn't want
anyone to bother him.

No children.
No grown ups.
When your mama takes
a nap it is just as though
she has gone into
her own little house and
shut the windows and doors.

These simple stories help children to see the outside world in different ways, to recognize the different needs of other people – such as the need for personal time and space – while also safely exploring and developing the inner world of the imagination.

Many children's stories are told in poetic form. In earlier chapters we discussed the importance of the music of language, something poems naturally do with sound; but poems also paint pictures with words and explore complex ideas. The poems written by William Blake in the eighteenth century still have resonance today, even though Blake was rejected as a madman by eighteenth-century society. Much of his writing focuses on opposing ideas such as heaven and hell, innocence and experience, spirit and reason, and the classic struggle of good and evil. Blake infused his writing not only with visionary imagination but also passion and detailed observation of the natural world. The visionary and child share a number of things in common – belief in things that cannot be scientifically explained in the physical world and the ability to see and hear things that are either beyond or simply by-pass others' conscious awareness. Whilst visions and mystical* experiences can be explained away by sceptics, the ability to form pictures and connections in the mind are essential elements of creativity and mental growth. Children may often respond naturally and intuitively to poems that share their fresh or visionary perception, such as this one – which is perhaps suitable for a very young child.

---

* Mysticism can be defined as an altered state of consciousness. But it is not merely a psychological state. If we trust the reports, the mystic state is filled with real, though not physical knowledge. The core of the mystic experience consistently reported is the sense of an identity between the deepest part of the self, and the creative force in all that exists, which one might term 'the divine'.

The Lamb
by William Blake[5]

Little Lamb, who made thee?
Dost thou know who made thee?
Gave thee life, & bid thee feed
By the stream & o'er the mead;
Gave thee clothing of delight,
Softest clothing, woolly, bright;
Gave thee such a tender voice,
Making all the vales rejoice?
Little Lamb, who made thee?
Dost thou know who made thee?
Little Lamb, I'll tell thee,
Little Lamb, I'll tell thee,
He is callèd by thy name,
For he calls himself a Lamb.
He is meek, & he is mild;
He became a little child.
I a child, & thou a lamb,
We are callèd by his name.
Little Lamb, God bless thee!
Little Lamb, God bless thee!

Other poems may be written from a child's perspective, articulating what the child may know emotionally but has not been able to put into words. This one, for example, for older children:

Children's Song
by R. S. Thomas

We live in our own world,
A world that is too small
For you to enter
Even on hands and knees,
The adult subterfuge.
And though you probe and pry
With analytic eye,

And eavesdrop all our talk
With an amused look,
You cannot find the centre
Where we dance, where we play,
Where life is still asleep
Under the closed flower,
Under the smooth shell
Of eggs in the cupped nest
That mock the faded blue
Of your remoter heaven.

As a small child I was certainly aware that 'my' world was different
from my parents' world and the world of my teachers and other
adults; that I could see, smell and hear things which they did not
notice. Use of advanced language as in this poem does not necessarily
prevent understanding of the underlying meaning. I think that even
quite young children can understand the idea that they have a private
(sensory) world, which is different from adults.

In 1929 the writer and poet John Drinkwater wrote an anthology,
More About Me,[6] which explored different aspects of childhood, also
largely written from a child's point of view. I loved these poems when
I was young and many of them are still as relevant for children today
as they were when they were written more than eighty years ago.
The first example below, which describes the difficulties involved in
learning multiplication tables, is timeless.

Multiplication

'Multiplication is vexation'
That is a thing they said,
And from twice times ten to ten times ten
It bothers me in my head.
I can do quite well if I'm told to tell
The whole of a table through,
But dodging about quite puts me out
Till I don't know what to do.
When seven times five are thirty-five
I can tell you seven times six,

But seven times eight must kindly wait,
Or get me into a mix.
And yes, if you please, in the middle of threes
They asked me eleven elevens,
And that is the kind that makes my mind
All at sixes and sevens.

Wanda Wild

Now Wanda Wild was not a child
That I could recommend;
She broke the rules in all her schools
Because they wouldn't bend;
She told her Aunt I shall I shan't,
And pulled the puppies tails,
She rang the bell and didn't tell,
And bit her finger nails.

She made a noise with several toys,
And if her mother said-
'Now Wanda will you please be still,'
She made some more instead;
She'd point and stare; she didn't care;
She trespassed in the wood;
She poured the ink all down the sink;
In fact, she wasn't good.

And sometimes if she took a tiff,
Although her nurse* was charming,
She stamped the floor, and banged the door,
And carried on alarming;
When told to wash she said 'O bosh!'
And took the soap and threw it
And broke a glass, and bold as brass
Then said she didn't do it.

---

*   Today the term nanny, au pair or child minder would be substituted for 'nurse'.

And, if you please, on days like these
She simply would not dress;
Till stitch by stitch they made her, which
Displeased her none the less,
And then she'd shout 'I won't go out,
Because I do not choose;
I do declare, I will not wear,
I *will* not wear my shoes.'

So you'll agree I think with me
That little Wanda Wild
Was not at all what we should call
A satisfactory child.
But, just between ourselves I mean,
I'm willing to explain
That you would look outside this book
For Wanda Wild in vain

Today Wanda Wild, like her predecessor Fidgety Phil, might easily be labelled as having a conduct disorder or Attention Deficit Hyperactivity Disorder (ADHD)! If her behaviour continued into later childhood and adolescence, in the first decade of the twenty-first century she might have been in line for an anti-social behaviour order (ASBO); but this poem reminds us that wilfulness, obstinacy and disobedience have been a normal part of childhood for generations, and it is the responsibility of parents and society to regulate and weave these personality traits into acceptable and positive behaviour. Almost every child knows what it feels like to be Wanda Wild, and can see the difference between behaving like her and *wanting* to behave like her. This sets the scene for starting to understand self-control. The stories in 'My Naughty Little Sister' and the behaviour of Beatrix Potter's Tom Kitten do much the same thing, not through sterile and direct teaching of right and wrong, but by using humour to tell stories which exaggerate aspects of behaviour. Caricature and comedy are often more powerful agents of learning than formal education.

Fairytales

Fairytales are not the property of childhood alone but are in a sense the archetypal form of oral narrative upon which so much 'literary' writing is based. Some of the best stories enjoyed by adults fall within the fairytale format. Features of fairy tales are that they usually involving legendary or magical deeds and creatures, are highly fanciful and often contain a hidden moral or explanation. They can be found throughout Europe and in many parts of Asia and many probably derive from folktales passed on as oral entertainment. Many of the best-loved fairytales today such as Cinderella, Bluebeard, Sleeping Beauty, Puss in Boots, Beauty and the Beast, The Frog Prince, Red Riding Hood, Snow White, Rumpelstiltskin, Rapunzel, The Tinder Box, and The Little Mermaid have been 'imported' from other parts of Europe and have been absorbed into English culture. Other more exotic tales such as the *Arabian Nights* and Aladdin came from further afield, notably Arabia. Traditional English fairy tales include Jack and the Beanstalk and Tom Thumb but the majority of fairytale texts recorded in Britain were found either in Scotland, Wales or among gypsy storytellers.

As only a few of these tales actually include fairies, they have some times been referred to as 'Wonder Tales' or 'Magic Tales'. The modern word 'fairy' derives from the French 'faerie', which meant 'enchantment' or 'magic', which in turn derived from 'fae', the source of the English word 'fay'. Both words originate from the Latin plural *fata,* used to personify the Fates, three goddesses who in ancient mythology governed human destiny. Thus, fairy stories are as much about human destiny and our encounters with 'enchantment' and good and evil in our search for meaning as they are about fairies. In the introduction to his book *The Uses of Enchantment: The Meaning and Importance of Tales of Magic and Wonderment,* the Austrian psycho-analyst Bettelheim writes:

> If we hope to live not just from moment to moment, but in true consciousness of our existence, then our greatest need and most difficult achievement is to find meaning in out lives [...] An understanding of the meaning of one's life is not suddenly acquired at a particular age, not even when one has reached

chronological maturity. On the contrary, gaining a secure understanding of what the meaning of one's life may or ought to be is what constitutes having attained psychological maturity.

The enchanted world of fairies and stepmothers, its magic forests and wise old kings, has been an integral part of childhood for hundreds of years. By revealing the true content of such stories, Bettelheim shows how children may make use of them to cope with baffling emotions, whether they be feelings of smallness and helplessness or the anxieties the child feels about strangers and the mysteries of the outside world. Taking the best-known stories in turn, he demonstrates how they work, consciously or unconsciously, to support and free the child.

One of the key features of fairytales is that they are fanciful in nature – meaning imagination or fantasy superficially exercised in a capricious manner (although the patterns, repetitions and rhythms in fairytales often, in fact, draw deeply on inherently human aspects of experience). As in poetry or drawing, fairytales nurture an artistic ability to create imagery and decorative detail which act as outer 'clothing' for deeper meaning. They are valuable because they contain an imaginative power that, like dream, can reach deeper than logic. Interestingly, as the popularity of fairytales in a younger generation of parents made wary by political correctness has declined, so have some of the words and sayings which accept fantasy as an inherent and valuable part of everyday existence. One of my father's favourite replies when told something new was, 'Well, fancy', meaning 'just imagine that'.

Just as night-dreaming is essential for mental health, so day-dreaming is important in helping to solve new problems and knit new information into the existing fabric of the known world. In following flights of fancy (fantasy) in the waking world, both children and adults are able to 'develop inner resources, so that one's emotions, imagination and intellect mutually support and enrich one another.'[7] More importantly, fairytales enable children to do this at different ages at whatever level or phase they are in at the time.

In one of my previous books, *What Babies and Children Really Need*,[8] I discussed how modern technological society – and childhood in particular – has become 'sanitized' in the sense that natural biological rhythms of life are held at one remove. In less complex cultures, as part of normal everyday living, children witness birth, breastfeeding, rites of passage, the killing and preparation of animals for food or clothing etc., inclusion of the aged and infirm within the family, death and burial ceremonies. These natural events are not hidden away in hospitals, abattoirs, nursing homes, morgues and chapels of rest. Children grow up understanding that life is not always easy or fair, but naturally brings with it joy and sadness, love and loss, growth and degeneration; and that every physical process has appropriate accompanying emotions. If as parents or society we seek to protect children from all unpleasant events, we do not equip them to deal with the real world. Paradoxically, one potential consequence of this type of over-protectiveness is a subsequent *in*crease in mental illness when children have to fit into the real world but lack the emotional tools, imagination or resilience to deal with it.

In 2009, a poll of 3,000 British parents carried out by TheBabyWebsite.com revealed that a quarter of mothers rejected some classic fairy tales saying that traditional fairytales were too scary and not politically correct enough. Stories that have been favourites with children for generations such as Snow White and the Seven Dwarfs, Cinderella, and Rapunzel, were being dropped by some families who thought they might emotionally damage their children:

> A third of parents refused to read Little Red Riding Hood because she walks through woods alone and finds her grandmother eaten by a wolf. One in ten said Snow White should be re-named because 'the dwarf reference is not PC'. Rapunzel was considered 'too dark' and Cinderella has been dumped amid fears she is treated like a slave and forced to do all the housework.[9]

Fairytales are important precisely because, among other things, they use 'make-believe' to teach fundamental principles of moral behaviour. Stereotypes of good and evil are used to illustrate that goodness endures and bad behaviour will eventually receive its just deserts. Far from demonizing the dwarfs, the story of Snow White shows that underlying physical diversity there can be greater kindness and generosity than is found in the stereotypes of beauty and wealth so lauded by celebrity-worshipping cultures. In many fairy stories

(Goldilocks for example), the smallest and weakest in the group is the one with whom the heroine identifies; and in The Emperor's New Clothes, vanity and pride are revealed as vacuous posturing without substance, masking stupidity and obstructing the use of common sense. These stories are not cruel and discriminatory; rather they help children to understand, firstly, the quirks and weaknesses of human behaviour in general, and secondly, to accept many of their own fears and emotions. As Bettelheim said:

> In child or adult, the unconscious is a powerful determinant of behavior. When the unconscious is repressed and its content denied entrance into awareness, then eventually the person's conscious mind will be partially overwhelmed by derivatives of these unconscious elements, or else he is forced to keep such rigid, compulsive control over them that his personality may become severely crippled [...] The prevalent parental belief is that a child must be diverted from what troubles him most: his formless, nameless anxieties, and his chaotic, angry, and even violent fantasies. Many parents believe that only conscious reality or pleasant and wish-fulfilling images should be presented to the child – that he should be exposed only to the sunny side of things. But such one-sided fare nourishes the mind only in a one-sided way, and real life is not all sunny.[10]

It is often said that the world is different for each generation and therefore we should not apply the standards of previous generations to the next. Actually, the natural, physical world changes very little, but the activities of mankind and society force accelerated social and evolutionary adaptations on each new generation.* I am always fascinated when I look through old photos. One of the first things I notice is how different things and fashions look from those of

---

*   When visiting a Steiner-Waldorf school recently, I was struck by how the faces of children who do not use e-media and are not forced into reading and writing before they are ready, still have a 'look' of faces I remember from when I was a child fifty years ago. Their faces, strikingly, looked free of tension. Conversely, a cosmetic surgeon recently commented on the ageing effects of computer use on women, suggesting that the need to focus at this visual distance for long periods of time is resulting in the formation of lines and jowls!

today; but if I peer a little further into the background of the picture, other than man-made structures the landscape has usually changed remarkably little. It is *human* nature that engages in often superficial change, yet keeps meeting, in different forms, the problems of greed, jealousy, anger and so on. Interestingly, most fairytales in some way incorporate these concepts, allowing children to externalize and thus acknowledge 'bad' feelings without guilt. Fairytales inevitably enlist children's innate wish for good to triumph. Many qualities embodied in these folktales parallel the Christian concept of the seven deadly sins and virtues.

Deadly sin	Opposing virtue
Pride	Humility
Avarice (greed)	Generosity
Envy	Love
Wrath (anger)	Kindness
Lust	Self-control
Gluttony	Temperance
Sloth (apathy or laziness)	Zeal

C. S. Lewis's much-loved tales of Narnia have enjoyed a resurgence of popularity in recent years. Their author was a professor of medieval literature and a late convert to Christianity, and these stories not only incorporate the seven deadly sins and opposing virtues in the behaviour of various characters, but also allegorize sacrifice, resurrection and a totalitarian regime. In one of the later chronicles, *The Horse and His Boy*, he introduces the hypothesis that all religions are fundamentally one and that the benevolent intentions of all faiths are received by a single deity while malevolent intentions are directed to a mythical demon similar to the concept of the devil. The Chronicles of Narnia are stories which can be enjoyed at many levels: simply as exciting adventure stories, but also, at their best, capable of revealing more profound beliefs, theories and universal truths. At some places, their allegorical meanings are evident just below the surface of the narrative, whereas true fairytales, as Betteheim indicates, admit of many different levels and interpretations, and can be understood by each person at their particular developmental and intellectual level. It may well be that in our more intellectual age it is hard to write fairytales that have the multi-layered depths acquired in an oral tradition deepened by each successive teller through the generations – all the more reason, therefore, to value them as a repository of archetypes that can scarcely be bettered.

Cinderella

The story of Cinderella includes many of the so-called sins and virtues: the good father who loses interest in his young child when his wife dies, and brings a new woman and her two daughters into the household, giving them the authority of stepmother and older sisters over his natural child; the younger child whose early life was so surrounded by love and affection that she does not immediately approach her new family with animosity, believing in the innate 'goodness' of others. She is ill-equipped to understand the envy, avarice, sloth and duplicity of her stepmother and older sisters. The relative virtue of the 'youngest child' is a theme in many fairytales, mirroring the relative powerlessness of the young child in a world where everyone else seems to be bigger, stronger and to know more of the world than she does. One of the morals of the story is that being small and less 'worldly wise' is only a temporary state. (There are many other possible interpretations – for instance that Cinderella as an aspect of ourselves we suppress but that will eventually, after many travails, come into rightful self-possession.)

Cinderella's sisters make her into a drudge who must answer their every whim. Their vanity knows no bounds, although by all accounts they have little to be proud of in this respect. When an invitation to the prince's ball arrives and Cinderella knows that she will not be able to go, her humiliation is complete when she is made to dress them for the ball. She is left feeling desolate, abandoned by those she loved.

The arrival of her fairy godmother is like the gift of opportunity and has many parallels in other cultures and stories, from the genii of the Arabian Nights, to the leprechauns in Irish literature and even the concept of a guardian angel – each 'agent for good' bringing material form to the heart's desire, or more importantly the potential to fulfil it. The transformation of mice into carriage horses, a pumpkin into a coach and rags into the most beautiful dress is perfectly possible in the magical thinking of a child's mind, or perhaps even the 'dream logic' of a sleeping adult, but there is also a stern warning that accompanies the magic. 'You must leave the ball before the clock strikes twelve. Disobey me and your wonderful dress will turn to rags. There will be no fine coach awaiting you; only an old pumpkin and four little mice. Do you understand?' The concept of obedience to a higher authority, which has provided the gift of opportunity, is part of the deal.

At the ball, all of Cinderella's virtues shine through. For a few hours, she is everything she is meant to be and she meets the prince of her dreams; but caught up in the joy and wonder of the evening she nearly forgets the warning of her fairy godmother. As the clock starts to strike, she runs away in haste, her dress turning to rags – but not before she loses one of her glass slippers in her flight down the stairs. She rushes home in rags, her carriage having turned back into a forlorn pumpkin at the palace gates, believing that she will never see her prince again. Her moment of opportunity was like a wonderful dream which fades with the coming of the day.

But, something from her dream has remained; something which retains its form and which, unbeknown to her, will lead her back to the land of opportunity. The glass slipper left behind on the stairs is found and given to the prince who cannot understand why his love deserted him. The prince's desire to find her again is so strong that he commands every woman in the land to try on the slipper until a perfect fit is found. When the stewards carrying the glass slipper arrive at Cinderella's house, she is pushed aside by the two older sisters, who struggle to squeeze their oversized feet into the dainty shoe. The steward notices Cinderella in the shadows and remembering the prince's stricture that every woman in the land should try the slipper, he insists that she must also try it. The slipper, is of course, a perfect fit because the shoe was made for Cinderella and Cinderella alone. No one else could take her place.

As she is taken to the palace to marry her prince, to live 'happily every after', the listener has learned of avarice, greed, envy, deceitfulness, cruelty, neglect and adult weakness on the part of the father, but also humility, generosity, love, kindness, obedience, zeal in the pursuit of opportunity, and most of all, of hope. The story is complete. It needs no explanation. The images speak for themselves in the child's mind, without need to intellectually 'point up' any single moral.

Some of C.S. Lewis's less well-known science-fiction novels are also a form of fairytale for older readers. *Out of the Silent Planet* is the first novel of a trilogy sometimes referred to as 'The Space Trilogy', which according to C.S. Lewis's biographer A.N. Wilson was written following a conversation between Lewis and J.R.R. Tolkien, in which both lamented the state of contemporary fiction. It was agreed that Lewis would write a space-travel story and Tolkien one based on time-travel.

In *Out of the Silent Planet* there is a moment when the hero, Professor Ransom – who dreams he visits the planet Malacandra – has spent so much time on Malacandra that when he sees his own kind in the distance, he does not recognize them as human beings. For the first time he views humans with the eyes of an outsider and mistakes them for clumsy aliens. This is a profound and shocking revelation, and reminds the reader that individual perception is highly subjective, and that others do not necessarily see the world in the same that we do – an important insight when taking the needs, perceptions and opinions of others into account. A later approach to this theme appears, for instance, in the 'Martian' poems of Craige Raine (specifically 'A Martian Sends a Postcard Home') which take a new look at human life and artefacts from a strange, alien perspective.

Many fairytales enable children to face their fears in imaginative form and, at least during the story, to overcome them. This is the general 'good overcomes evil' or 'smallest or derided wins in the end' theme, which runs through a great many traditional fairytales. Snow White and the Seven Dwarfs, The Sleeping Beauty and The Ugly Duckling are all examples of this.

The Ugly Duckling

When the Ugly Duckling is born, his mother looks at him in alarm and says, '*What* are you? I hope you're not a turkey child. I just couldn't bear that kind of disappointment.' His siblings ask him why he isn't pretty like them, and the description of his silence and an unhappy feeling descending on him like a damp mist is something every child has felt at some time. Fear of not being good enough, of not being loved, of not 'fitting in', of being abandoned, misunderstood; or of the world not being fair – all of these fears are a normal part of growing up, but children do not know that these (we hope) fleeting episodes will pass. Anticipatory fear in the absence of real and present danger is a form of fantasy – a projection of how we think we are viewed by others and what *might* happen in the future.

As Mother Duck reluctantly accepts him as part of her family, she is constantly checking to see if he really is one of them. He can swim so he cannot be a turkey after all, but she readily accepts the cloak of shame when others laugh at him. Unable to bear it any longer, the ugly duckling sets out to find his happiness. He meets the same attitudes outside of his adoptive family. He is too ugly to be befriended by the geese, too bedraggled to be eaten by the dogs; an old woman takes pity on him, but when she finds he cannot even lay an egg or cluck like her hen he is chased away by her cat. All his worst fears are confirmed. He does not belong. He nearly dies as he struggles to survive alone through the long, hard winter, and when spring comes at last he sees some beautiful white birds on the lake. As the ice melts he sees a reflection in the water and the reflection reveals not the ugly scarecrow that he had expected, but a graceful, long-necked swan; and the beautiful white birds welcome him into their family. The ugly duckling knows for the first time what it is to be happy. He has found his true family at last.

Inside the wan, little ugly duckling, with all his fears and isolation, the swan was present and waiting all the time. The transformation to a creature of beauty is not the main point of the story, although the symbolism serves a purpose. The story explores many human emotions from fear, rejection, enforced conformity, discrimination, ignorance, shame and loneliness to endurance, hope, growth, maturity and the courage to be true to the self. Although beauty may serve as the passport, it is belonging which is the ultimate prize.

The Water Babies

Charles Kingsley's *Water Babies* tells a different sort of story of the journey from savage behaviour born of ignorance to success acquired through knowledge and experience. Set in Victorian times, it tells the story of Tom, a child chimney sweep, who escapes a dreadful life by being transformed into a water baby by the Queen of the Fairies. The story follows his journey to redemption, starting as an ignorant boy, who is the product of the cruel upbringing he has received from his master Mr. Grimes. Throughout his journey, better ways of behaving are inferred through the characters that he meets along the way – the indubitable Mrs Be-done-by-as-you-did and Mrs Do-as-you-would-be-done-by – being examples of this. The story also has mythological elements and contains some wonderful natural descriptions. As with anything really well written, it takes the reader beyond the mundane, leading us in the author's footsteps in observing aspects of the world and our place within it. It goes on to warn that any journey of discovery or success is not without risk or failure along the way, pointing out that, '… people who make up their minds to go and see the world as Tom did, must needs find it a weary journey. Lucky for them if they do not lose heart and stop half way, instead of going bravely to the end as Tom did.[11]

As I have suggested, fairytales are not just for children. The following story, *When Two Hearts Were One*, originally written by my husband Peter Blythe when he was a young sailor returning from in Ceylon at the end of the second world war, and rewritten in 2010 to be included in this book, is a fairy story for adults.

When Two Hearts Were One
by Peter Blythe (1945)[12]

Before we are born we are filled with an inner sense of happiness, well-being and completeness. We really are complete.

In this 'other place', which we inhabit before we are born, we have two eyes with which to see the glorious things around us, and there are a lot of wondrous things to see because we are in a realm of beauty. We have two nostrils to enjoy all the delicate smells always around us. We have a mouth with which to eat and tongue to taste all the flavours of the surrounding world. We have two lungs so we can breathe and fill our being with the spirit of the air. We have two arms to hold things and to give us balance and we have two legs which give us the freedom to move around the wonderful world we are in. But most of all we have two hearts that beat as one.

There are no men and women, boys and girls, male or female – just us – a complete us.

Our life in our first world is beyond human description. Our life is full of all-encompassing love. Everywhere there are the most beautiful colours; gentle scents swirl around us causing us to inhale deeply very often. There is no strife, anger, fear, anxiety, envy, greed, jealousy, illness or death. We are all a part of each other, attached by an invisible connection. Everything we need is there for us whenever we want something, so crime is unknown.

We were complete in every sense.

Then the Creator felt we, his creations, needed something more. So, for a long time He pondered the question, 'What shall I do?' Then He knew what should be done.

He decided we needed to strive to find love and happiness instead of it being a divine gift, but his answer gave rise to another question, 'How shall I do this?'

Time passed and then He knew what to do.

He would separate us; but before he put His plan into operation He decided He would create another 'world' which was quite different from our Home-World. And it took time before our new world was ready to receive us. While the Creator fashioned our new world we continued to live in blissful ignorance.

Then He separated 'us' and sent each one to live in our new world. Each part of the 'us' he sent to live in the new world, were placed many, many miles apart, and in his divine wisdom we were 'born' nearly complete. We had two halves in our brain, two eyes, two nostrils, two lungs, two arms, and two legs, but only one heart. We were incomplete.

Then the Creator showed his brilliance: he placed the heart from 'us' into a woman and the other heart into a man. So from the moment we are 'born' we know, we feel, we are incomplete.

Slowly but surely the 'us' from our real world are 'born' in our new world, but from the moment of our birth we look for our other heart so we can become complete again.

When we are very tiny, a new-born baby, we feel our mother is the other part of us. We recognise her heartbeat when we are placed on her breast because we heard it for the last nine months as we prepared for our new world. And then we get our first shock: our mother's heart is not our other, missing heart; only for a short time we knew love and togetherness once again. Then we are alone.

When we go to school, without realizing it, we are searching for our other heart. That is why we find ourselves drawn to a girl in our class. More often than not she is not our heart, but there was something which seemed familiar and as a result attracted us to her

Our next stage in our new world is to give up our search for our other heart. It is far too painful and we go through the stage where we tell the boys in our classes that we consider girls to be 'silly', 'they are not like us'; but even as we say this we notice certain girls who we would like to know better.

All this begins to alter when we go to senior school and we become definitely interested in finding 'the right girl to be our girl-friend' and sometimes the girl, looking for her other heart, is equally attracted to us. We are in love and everything in this world changes. We begin to recapture the wonderful feelings that were ours before we were born, when we had two hearts. But all too often the girl we love is not our other heart or she decides that we are not her heart and we separate. Then we feel desolate, lost or heart-broken. And worse still, this may happen many times in our life on this earth as we grow up and into adulthood. But all is not lost.

Each time we fall in love the person we love gives us something, even if the break-up has been agonising. It might be a new way of smiling, a joy in nature, a new way of looking at the trees or the sky; a new pleasure in reading certain types of books, an entirely new way of enjoying listening to music or certain pieces of music or a new interest in art. Or it may be something so small that we only recall it quite infrequently, but everyone who has been in love gives something to the one who has been loved.

And if we are very, very lucky we will meet our other heart somewhere. The moment of meeting is magical. It is as if we have known each other all our lives. We don't fall in love with each other. From the very moment we meet there is love between us, and when we speak to each other for the first time it feels as if we are starting in the middle of something we have talked about before. There is shared laughter and 'our' own sense of humour. We recapture all the things we had before we were born; all the things we had when we had two hearts.

But what happens if you don't meet your other heart? What happens if your other heart dies before you do?

Do not despair. When we die and return to our other world, our other heart will either be there waiting for us if death has separated us, so we can know the complete and total love of being one once again. Or if we never meet our other heart in this other, all is not lost. When we die our other heart will find us and make us complete once again.

A fairytale? Of course not!

Fables

While fairy stories usually contain a hidden moral, one of their enduring charms is that they have a happy ending. Fables on the other hand contain a moral message, but do not necessarily end well. Certain of Aesop's fables such as *The Boy who Cried Wolf* and *The Tortoise and the Hare* are well known, and the moral of the tale is so familiar that the title of story alone is sufficient to 'tell the moral tale'. Each of the fables carries a warning and is short enough to be enjoyed by even young children if told as a bedtime story.

The Ass, the Fox and The Lion
Aesop's Fables[13]

An ass and a fox went into partnership and sallied out to forage for food together. They hadn't gone far before they saw a lion coming their way, at which they were both dreadfully frightened. But the fox thought he saw a way of saving his own skin, and went boldly up to the lion and whispered in his ear, 'I'll manage that you shall get hold of the ass without the trouble of stalking him, if you'll promise to let me go free.' The lion agreed to this, and the fox then rejoined his companion and contrived before long to lead him by a hidden pit, which some hunter had dug as a trap for wild animals, and into which he fell. When the lion saw that the ass was safely caught and couldn't get away, it was to the fox that he first turned his attention, and he soon finished , and then at his leisure proceeded to feast upon the ass.

The moral of the story is clear: that if you betray a friend the act of betrayal will backfire on you, and it is you who will be destroyed by your own act of betrayal. Children do not actually need this explained to them. The story is sufficient unto itself. As opposed to factual stories or the direct teaching of codes of behaviour through instruction and punishment, fairytales and fables both entertain and teach:

> Their special genius is that they do so in terms which speak directly to children [...] The way that 'true' stories unfold is as alien to the way the pre-pubertal child's mind functions as the supernatural events of the fairytale are to the way the mature intellect comprehends the world. Strictly realistic stories run counter to the child's inner experiences, he will listen to them and maybe get something out of them, but he cannot extract much personal meaning from them that transcends obvious content [...] When realistic stories are combined with ample and psychologically correct exposure to fairytales, then the child receives information which speaks to both parts of his budding personality – the rational and the emotional.[14]

One example where this does not occur is in children with autism, who can often understand a limited range of facts, but find it difficult to enter the fantasy world of fairytales or extrapolate the moral of a fable.

Fables, like fairytales, can be written for all ages and stages of life. C.S. Lewis's *The Screwtape Letters,* first published in book form in 1942 is essentially a fable for grown-ups. The story takes the form of a series of letters from a senior demon, Screwtape, to his nephew, a junior tempter named Wormwood, giving him advice on the most effective methods of securing the damnation of a British man, known only as 'the Patient'. Screwtape is not obviously demonic. Instead, he teaches Wormwood how best to manipulate all of the human weaknesses, offering him detailed advice on various methods of undermining faith and promoting sin. Both senior and junior demon live in a peculiarly topsy-turvy world in moral terms, where individual benefit and greed are seen as the greatest good. These letters have parallels not only in Christian teaching but also in the behaviour of individuals, society and governments. The letters are fictitious precursors of the modern concept of 'spin'. The truth can be turned to serve any purpose, the greatest deception of all being self-deception.

The most enduring stories can be understood at many levels. Even some of the oldest biblical stories such as the story of creation in Genesis fulfill this requirement. Some people believe that the world was literally created by God in seven days; others adamantly refute the concept of God or a higher being having any part in the creation of the universe, using scientific conjectures to explain the origins of the universe and the evolution of all matter and living things. But religion and science do not *have* to be mutually exclusive, and the story of creation can also be viewed as an allegory – a way of explaining evolution in the light of what was known at the time.

All matter and forms of life are the product of energy. Whether you believe in nature, the Big Bang, or divine creation as the hand or force behind it, in the beginning there must have been an original source of *energy*. Energy is expressed through movement, from the motion of the planets to the movement of the tides and the whispering of the wind in the trees. Einstein observed that all forms of life share the characteristic of motion, and that even matter is movement frozen in time. Time itself is the product of space and movement through space. In Genesis we are told that God created the world and mankind in seven days. The theory of evolution explains in detail how the world has developed increasingly complex forms of life and matter over millions of years, but if the *time* factor is removed from the argument, then the sequence of creation and evolution follow a similar pattern: beginning with light, then night and day, water and air, sea and earth, creatures of the sea, air and land, and finally mankind.

These diverse ways of explaining complex ideas and developments are similar to the ways in which the two sides of the human brain process information in different ways – the right brain processing information visually, holistically and intuitively, and largely uncon-cerned with rigid timeframes in its need to understand the whole, while the left brain is more logical, and analytical, pays attention to detail, and needs to support what it sees and feels with evidence. While both sides of the brain develop throughout childhood, in the early years of life, the right brain matures slightly in advance of the left hemisphere,[15] and plays a more dominant role in processing expression and regulation of emotional information:[16]

> It has been suggested that investigations into the neural bases for social interaction should focus on the role of the holistic, affec-tive, silent right hemisphere in the mediation of social life.[17]

> The right brain also has more neurological connections in a down-ward direction to centres involved in the experience of emotions, feelings and instinctual reactions to the outside world.[18]

When new information is experienced with emotion, it tends to be remembered:

> The right-holistic mode is particularly good at grasping patterns of relations between the component parts of a stimulus array, integrating many inputs simultaneously to eventually arrive at a complete configuration.[19]

It is also functions in

> a present-centredness or timeless experience in which all events are perceived to occur immediately and simultaneously. This style of thinking is reflected across many Eastern cultures where no distinction is made between past and present, and time is considered to be an ontological absurdity. The non-linear mode is cultivated deliberately in these eastern mystical traditions for the purpose of arriving at a more accurate picture of reality not based on time, linear consciousness, or the physical changes of this illusory world.[20]

Fairy stories – which traditionally begin with 'Once upon a time', 'Once, long ago', 'In old times, when wishing still helped' – place the story outside of 'real' time and space. Children are able to understand that these stories pertain to the 'real' or physical world yet unfold in a realm beyond it.

Bettelheim observed that 'The truth of fairy stories is the truth of our imagination, not that of normal causality. […] Before a child can come to grips with reality, he must have some frame of reference to evaluate it.'[21] When a child asks if a story is true, she wants to know if it contributes something to her understanding. In other words she wants to know which part of the story is relevant to *her*.

Some of the best teachers are those who convey information by telling stories. For many years my husband trained post-graduate students in the use of specific techniques which he had developed. One of his students complained that 'he is very entertaining, but he teaches *sideways*; each time he starts to tell us how to do something, or what the findings of a test mean, he goes off at a tangent and tells a story. My notes are all over the place, and I don't know how to start organizing them to put what I have learned into a structure'. While there are many different learning styles, from structured and linear to anecdotal, the telling of stories helps pupils to derive meaning from facts and to integrate new information into what is already known. At the end of a course, all of his students had not only acquired factual knowledge but deeper understanding of what they had learned and how to apply that knowledge to new situations – in other words, to think for themselves.

The parables of the New Testament provide examples of stories used in a similar way, to invite the listener to find her own meaning. In the context of the time (when the majority of the population were illiterate) the telling of stories was one of the primary mediums of education. 'The good teacher does not bid you enter the house of his wisdom, but rather leads you to the threshold of your own mind.'[22]

The telling of stories encourages the formation of pictures in the mind's eye, as words are translated into images and information is woven into our inner world. The use of Guided Affective Imagery (GAI) serves as an example of how powerful this process can be.

GAI is a form of therapy developed by Hans Leuner, in which the patient is asked to close his eyes and make a journey under the guidance of the therapist. The story may go something like this:

> 'I want you to imagine a country lane. On one side of the country lane is a gate which leads you into the field. I want you to go through the gate and tell me what you see …'

> The patient may describe a field or enclosed space. The patient is asked,

> 'Is there another way out of the space, other than the way you came in?'

> If the patient says, yes, then he is instructed to go out of the space and follow where the way takes him.

> The way may lead down to a stream. The patient is asked whether he would like to follow the stream up towards the source or down towards the outlet. The direction the patient chooses is not important. What matters is what he describes along the way. On reaching a destination he is invited to stop and rest for a while. When ready, he will be instructed to turn around and retrace his steps back to the beginning, describing what he sees on the return journey.

No analysis of the journey is required. Often, the process of *making* the journey brings about change, and just as we all know that scenery looks different depending on which direction we are travelling in, so the process of setting out and returning seems to bring about beneficial emotional and cognitive change.

> The power of the imagination for growth and healing is still little understood, but may be one of the most potent elements of fairytales and fables for children's emotional and social development. By enriching children's imagination, fairy tales provide new solutions to the dilemmas of childhood through continually reworking and developing ruminative fantasies and daydreams such that mastery over childhood problems can be achieved.[23]

The German philosopher, poet, historian and playwright Friederich von Schiller wrote in his *The Aesthetic Education of Man*:

Deeper meaning resides in the fairytales told me in my child-hood than in any truth that is taught in life.[24]

In a nutshell

- Reading and telling stories is sociable.
- Fairytales and fables are narratives told and retold orally from one group to another across generations and centuries. The stories usually contain 'collective wisdom' and imaginative archetypes acquired over time and across cultures.
- Fairytales and fables usually entertain and educate.
- They provide lessons in morality, cultural values and social requirements.
- They encourage imagination, fantasy and humour.
- They help all age groups to understand the human predicament.
- They allow for the examination and reframing of human problems.
- They help all ages to live with the 'unknowable'.
- Analysis and understanding of unconscious material.

Notes

1 H. Hoffman: *Struwwelpeter.* Dover Publications Inc., New York 1995.
2 R. Williams: 'Many parents failing to read to children, survey shows.' *The Guardian,* 30 April 2010.
3 M. Wise Brown: *Good Night Moon.* Macmillan Children's Books, London 2010.
4 B. Schenk de Regniers: *A Little House of My Own.* Collins Press, London 1961.
5 W. Blake: *Songs of Innocence* (1789) facsimile edition, Tate Publishing 2007.
6 J. Drinkwater: *More About Me.* C.W. Collins Sons and Co. Ltd., London 1929.
7 B. Bettlelheim. *The Use of Enchantment. The Meaning and Importance of Fairy Tales.* Penguin Books, London 1976.
8 S.A. Goddard Blythe: What Babies and Children Really Need. Hawthorn Press. Stroud 2008.
9 G. Paton: 'Traditional fairy tales not PC enough.' http://www.telegraph.co.uk/culture/books/4125664/Traditional-fairytales-not-PC-enough-for-parents.html
10 Bettelheim, op. cit.
11 C. Kingsley: *The Water Babies* (1863) Oxford University Press 1995.

12 P. Blythe: *Fairy Stories for Grown-Ups.* Unpublished manuscript.

13 *Aesops' Fables,* Translated by V.S. Vernon Jones. Wordsworth Classics, Ware 1994.

14 Bettlelheim, op. cit.

15 N. Geschwind, A.M. Galaburda: *Cerebral Lateralization: Biological Mechanisms, Associations, and Pathology.* The MIT Press, Boston 1987.

16 R. Joseph: 'The neuropsychology of development. Hemispheric laterality, limbic language and the origin of thought.' *Journal of Clinical Psychology.* 38: 4–33. 1982.

17 P.R Barchas and K.M. Perlaki: 'Processing of preconsciously acquired information measured by hemispheric asymmetry and selection accuracy. '*Behavioral Neuroscience.* 100: 343–9. 1986.

18 A. N. Schore: *Affect Regulation and the Origin of the Self. The Neurobiology of Emotional Development.* Lawrence Eerlbaum Associates Inc. Publishers. Hillsdale, New Jersey 1994.

19 J.F. Iaccino: *Left Brain – Right Brain Differences. Inquiries, evidence and new approaches.* Lawrence Erlbaum Associates Inc. Publishers. Hillsdale, New Jersey 1993.

20 D. Lee: 'Codification of reality. Lineal and non-lineal.' In RE Ornstein (ed.): *The Nature of Human Consciousness.* Viking Press, New York 1973.

21 Bettelheim op. cit.

22 K. Gibran: *The Prophet.* Heineman, London 1982.

23 H.C. Leuner: 'Guided affective imagery (GAI).' *American Journal of Psychotherapy.* 23/1.22 1969.

24 Quoted in: D.W. Chan: 'Stories and storytelling in teaching and child psychotherapy.' *CUHK Primary Education.* 3/2: 27–31, 1995.

CHAPTER 6

A Day in the Garden

A story for parents and children with suggested activities

The following story can be used in several ways:

1 As a bedtime story for children and parents to enjoy together.
2 A play activity for parents and child. The parent reads the story and as the child becomes familiar with the characters in the story, the child acts out the part of the characters.
3 A more structured daily activity for children from about age three, particularly if there are minor concerns about a child's balance or coordination development. The suggested exercises may be carried out every day for a period of up to 6 months.

Please note   If you have any concerns about your child's physical development, please check with your health visitor before carrying out any daily exercise programme. If your child is currently receiving treatment for a related disorder, check with your consulting physician before using any of the suggested exercises.

A New Day

All was quiet in the garden. Night had covered the flowers and creatures in a cloak of darkness. The flowers had curled up inside their petals to keep warm, and most of the creatures except Bertie the Badger and Mol the Owl (who both worked at night), were sound asleep.

As a chink of light started to rise in the distant sky, the birds began to chatter.

'Time to get up; time to get up; it's a beautiful day; the worms are out and it's time to play.'

'No time to sleep; can't stay still; too much to do; time to eat; come along, fly with me; come and greet the dawn; it's a bea—utiful day.'

As the birds swooped and sang at the joy of greeting a new day, the other inhabitants of the garden began to stir.

Dizzy the Daisy was a sun lover. Night time was alright because she could wrap her petals around herself into a warm blanket, disappear inside the covers and dream of following the sun in its path all day long; but when night started to slip away, she longed to see the sun again and did not like to wake up to a grey or dreary day.

Morning (wake-up) exercises

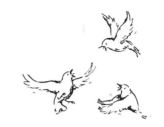

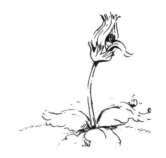

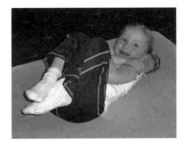

Lie on back with arms crossed, hands curled, resting on shoulders, knees bent and ankles crossed.

Slowly uncurl fingers and toes.
Pause.

As the light started to tickle her petals, she gingerly opened just one of them to feel if it was warm enough to come out. A drop of dew had collected on her leaf and she shivered to try to make it roll off. 'Atishoo—', she sneezed, as the cold morning air got up her nose, 'atishoo—' This time the dewdrop did fall to the ground and she started to feel a little warmer.

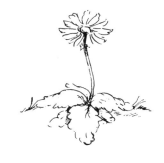

Curl fingers and toes.
Pause

Dizzy was very vain. She knew she was pretty but could never quite believe that other flowers in the garden were not more eye-catching than her. This meant that she always tried to be the first at everything, in the hope she would be noticed. This included making sure she was the first flower to flash her petals in the mornings.

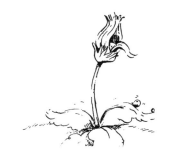

Dizzy's need to be noticed may have been because she was in fact quite small and one of a family of many daises on the lawn. Not that there was anything wrong with being a daisy, it was just that some of the bigger flowers such as Lupin and Dahlia seemed to attract more attention, much more admiration from passing bees, and showed off so.

Slowly, she opened out her petals one by one.

Slowly open out first the
fingers and then toes.
Uncross the arms and legs
and slowly open them out.
(Do not straighten the arms
and legs completely)

Daisy reasoned that being one very small flower amongst many others meant the only way to be noticed was to look her best at all times. She stre—tched out her petals (head and neck), turning to one side and then the other, as she tried to decide which way flattered her most. She fluttered her petals at Mr. Sun, who was beaming down at her from a small corner of the garden. Still not satisfied she thought, 'If only I was a little taller, not only could I get nearer to the sun but I would have a better view of the comings and goings in the garden.'

Slowly stretch the neck back (without straining).
Gently wave hands and feet as if wafting them in the air.

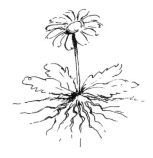

Stop waving hands and feet.

Making an enormous effort, she pushed her roots (toes) down as far as she could under the ground and spread her leaves (hands) as far out as they would go. This was hard work and she could only stretch herself this far for a second or two.

Stretch arms and hands, legs and feet as far as comfortable.

'Whooooooo—' she said, 'this morning workout is really tiring.'

Relax

She rested for a few moments before trying again. After the fifth time she stopped, feeling quite exhausted.

Curl and uncurl hands and feet a few times.

'Dear me', she thought, 'Dizzy you really are very unfit.'

By this time her roots and leaves were beginning to ache so much that she curled and squeezed them a few times, finally giving them a good shake before rearranging her petals so that they could best face the sun.

Shake hands and feet a few times.

'Dizzy my dear,' said Mr. Sun, 'there really is no need to go to so much trouble. Provided there are no clouds in the sky, I would shine on you in the morning anyway. The only time I can't see you is when the garden wall gets in the way as I move across the garden during the day. You are quite lovely, my dear, and there really is no need to make so much effort for me.'

Rest.

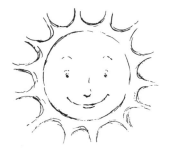

Dizzy felt her petals turn a deeper shade of pink at the edges as she blushed. Mr. Sun had not only noticed her, he had talked to her as well. Everyone knew that Mr. Sun was the King of the Garden, and it was he who decided whether it was warm or cold, night or day, how much you grew and whether you had a good breakfast or not. For a few moments, she was so overcome, she quite forgot to worry about how she looked, and stood with her mouth open in surprise.

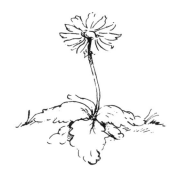

Dizzy also knew that if you made Mr. Sun cross he could make life very uncomfortable. Only once had she seen him angry. For a whole day he had blazed down on the garden, not allowing a cloud in the sky to pass in front of him. She and the other flowers had got hotter and hotter, more and more thirsty, and she had been so tired by the middle of the afternoon that she had not been able to keep her petals open until bedtime, letting them droop limply as she stood exhausted, longing for him to pass through the garden so she could rest in the shade of the garden wall. She did not know what had made him so fierce that day but she was clever enough to know that while it was wonderful to be noticed, she never wanted to do anything to make him angry again.

The birds had passed their first burst of excitement at the new day. Having swooped down to pick up grubs and the first worms of the morning for breakfast, they were now content to fly gently from bush to bush, hopping from leaf to leaf and gossiping amongst themselves.

Meanwhile,

Christopher the Caterpillar was asleep under a pile of leaves. Unlike the birds, who seemed to have boundless energy from the moment daylight appeared, Christopher was not a morning person. It took him a *long* time to wake up and he found the noise of the birds very tiresome.

He stre—tched a little, and then quickly curled up into a ball again.

'Too soon,' he thought, 'just another few minutes' sleep. If only those birds would be quiet.'

Just as he was settling into a lovely dream all about cabbage leaves and how good they tasted, something started to disturb his bed of leaves. Not only was it disturbing his bed, it was actually, walking all over it.

Daytime exercises

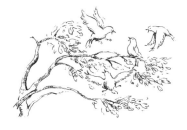

Lie on the tummy.

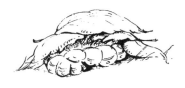

Curl up into a ball and then stretch out.

Repeat 2 or 3 times.

His first reaction was to curl up tighter into a ball in the hope that the uninvited guest would leave, but the visitor appeared to be making itself quite at home, scrabbling and burrowing at his bed.

'Bother,' he thought. 'I suppose I shall have to get up.'

'Has that dreadful din quietened down yet?'

'If it wasn't for those noisy flying things I would be able to sleep until noon every day. As it is, I have to get up long before I am ready, and I don't *like* it. What is it about this garden that some people get up when they feel like it, with no thought for anyone else? It really is most inconsiderate.'

This time, he lifted his head and neck up, to try to nudge his way through the bed of leaves and dislodge the unwanted visitor.

For a moment the visitor stopped scrabbling and stood perfectly still. When Christopher became still, the visitor started moving again.

'Would you *mind?*' said Christopher. 'It really is very rude to walk all over someone's bed when they are still sleeping in it.'

Curl up again.

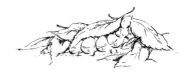

Lie on the tummy with legs straight, arms resting by the sides, head central, with upper body resting on the forearms.

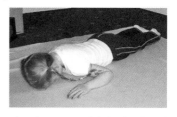

Slowly tip and lift the head up a little way until the back of the head is in line with the body.
Pause.

The visitor scuttled round in small circles, stirring the leaves into an untidy pile, right on the top of Christopher's head. Soon the bedding and visitor felt so heavy that he had to lower his head to the ground again.

Slowly lower the head to the ground so that the forehead is resting on the floor again.

'I say, this really is terribly rude. Would you please get *off*?' he mumbled with his face on the ground.

Rest.

'So sorry, so sorry. Oh dear. Oh dear, oh dear. How silly of me. Of course I will get off at once.'

Go up on to hands and knees.

The visitor was Wenna the Wood Louse, who was very well-intentioned but had the most dreadfully poor eyesight and was always bumping into things and getting in the way. This morning she had mistaken a pile of leaves with Christopher underneath it for a pile of twigs and had been trying to find her way with her feet. The more anxious she became, the faster she moved and the more flustered she got, losing any sense of direction and turning around in small circles.

Turn round twice in one direction.
Pause.
Close the eyes and stay still for 5 seconds.
Open eyes.
Turn round twice in the other direction.
Pause.
Staying on hands and knees, close eyes and stay still for 5 seconds.
Open eyes.

'For goodness sake, my dear, stop fussing and *think*', said Christopher.

'Oh yes, oh yes, of course, how sensible of you. All I have to do is stand still and I will be able to work out which way to go next'

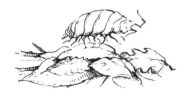

'Just don't stand there for too long. You are giving me a headache.'

'I won't be a moment, but I feel so giddy and I can't think which way to go.'

She started to turn around the other way, in the hope that she could undo her giddiness, but this was too much for Christopher.

Turn round once in each direction again, pausing for five seconds after each turn, with eyes closed.

'If you don't get off my bed this instant, I am going to arch my back and tip you off', he said.

Wenna was so alarmed that she stopped turning immediately and stood perfectly still, clinging to the remaining leaves with her toes. She knew from experience that if she was tipped on to her back she would get stuck like that and it might take her all day to roll over again.

Christopher bent his head down and arched his back.

Lying on the tummy, slowly bend the neck forwards and arch the back.

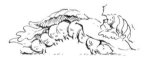

Wenna, who was clutching precariously on the falling pile of leaves with her toes, was frozen to the spot.

Christopher lifted his head and hollowed his back.

Slowly extend the neck and hollow the back

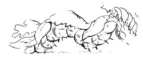

Wenna started to lose her grip.

Christopher arched and hollowed his back again.

Repeat the movements a little faster.

'Oooooh', cried Wenna, as she slowly tumbled off the pile of leaves, rolled over to land on a soft mound of earth and ended up lying on her back with her legs in the air.

Stop the movements and slowly roll over several times (as if rolling off a pile of pillows) until lying on back.

'Oh, this is so un*dignified*', she said.

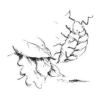

She turned her head from side to side to see if she could figure out the best way to roll over, but each time she turned her head, her arms and legs straightened on the same side, stopping her from rolling over.

Lie on back with head central, with arms and legs slightly bent. Slowly turn the head from side to side, straightening the arm and leg on the side to which the head is turned, but keeping the opposite arm and leg bent.

Wenna brought her head back to the middle and clapped her hands in agitation, trying to make her very little brain work harder to solve the problem.

Return the head to the centre and make small repeated clapping movements with the hands.

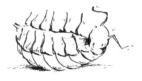

'There must be a way', she thought. She remembered that when she became anxious and flustered she could never think properly, so she lay calmly for a few moments, gazing at the canopy of trees beneath the sky as she tried to work out what to do next.

Lie still for a few seconds with the head central, feet on the floor, knees bent and arms slightly bent ('resting' position).

Next time, when she turned her head to one side, she stretched her fingers and tried to reach for a twig.

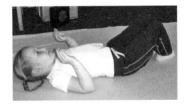

'If only I can grip the twig with my fingers, I can pull myself over', she thought, but however hard she tried, the twig remained just out of her reach. She tried to turn to the other side but the twigs were even further away.

Turn the head to one side, stretching the arm, fingers and leg on the same side only. Turn the head to the other side, stretching the arm, fingers and leg on the same side. Repeat 2 or 3 times. Return the head to the centre, feet on the floor, knees bent and arms bent (resting position)

She remembered that her father always used to tell her that her problem was she tried to do everything too fast, and if only she slowed down she would not be so clumsy.

Next time she turned her head as slowly as she could, and instead of reaching for the twig, she tucked her arm to the side of her body and brought the other arm and leg across. This time she started to feel herself turning.

'Not quite far enough', she thought, but no amount of pushing would make her roll any further.

She tried the same thing to the other side, but still could not turn quite far enough.

She returned to the middle and then started to rock from side to side. Each time she moved to one side a little further, until finally as she rocked to one side, arms and leg tucked in, she brought the other arm and leg across and her world started to move. For one moment everything was upside down, the next, she was back on her hands and feet again.

To her alarm, she found herself face to face with Christopher, and unable to bear any further scolding from him, she scuttled off into the undergrowth.

***Slowly** turn the head to one side but this time keep the arm and leg on the same side straight and tucked in to the body. Bend the arm and leg on the opposite side and bring them across the body to the midline of the body*

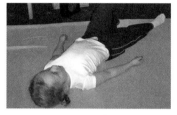

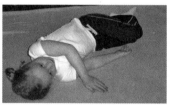

Return head, arms and legs to 'resting' position.
Repeat the movements on the other side.
Gently rock from side to side.
Repeat movements above from side to side, rocking gently until the body starts to roll over.

Christopher was ready for breakfast; and after all his early morning exercise had worked up quite an appetite. Normally he would have made his breakfast from local leaves, but feeling in need of something more substantial he started to work his way towards his favourite milkweed plant on the other side of the lawn.

Lie on the tummy.

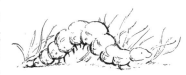

He lifted his head, stretched his neck, shrugged his shoulders and started to amble along the caterpillar trail by arching and hollowing his back and pushing with his feet. It took a long time and a lot of effort to go only a short way, but as he slithered onto the damp grass it was easier to glide along the surface. Mr. Sun was shining down, and by the time he reached the edge of the grass he was not only hungry and thirsty but also hot and tired.

Lift up the head.
Shrug and unshrug the shoulders.
Arch and hollow the back a few times.
Bed the toes into the ground and push off with the toes.

Using a combination of these movements, slowly move forwards.

He wriggled onto a patch of earth next to his favourite plant, Miss Milkweed, and for a few moments rested under the shade of her leaf. All he had to do now was climb up onto the leaf, and breakfast would be his.

(This is much easier if done on a slippery surface such as wood laminated floor).

This was easier said than done. First he had to lift up his head, neck and shoulders, using his arms to support his weight. Then, gripping the stalk with his fingers he had to pull himself up onto the stalk. Using a combination of pulling with his hands and walking with his feet, he climbed up the stem until he was resting on the leaf.

After a small distance. Stop.

Find a sturdy flat surface with which to make a short slide.
Slowly climb up the surface.

Once there he started to munch.

It had taken him so long to get up, to reach Miss Milkweed and climb up onto her leaf that it was now nearly lunchtime. He ate more than he had intended and started to feel quite sleepy.

'I had better not fall asleep here', he thought. 'I might fall off, or worse still get sun burned.'

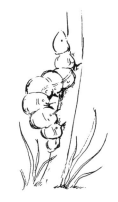

Slowly slide back down the surface, feet first.

It was nearing the middle of the day and Mr. Sun was doing a splendid job of keeping the garden warm. Christopher turned round so that he could go down feet first, slithering down Miss Milkweed's stalk. This was much easier and more fun than climbing up and he would have liked to have done it again.

Slowly he crawled back through the grass until he reached some shade. Hot and tired after his exercise, he shed some of his outer clothes and used them to form a hammock which he hung between two stems of a plant. Wearily he crawled in, and lay on his back; and as he gently swayed from side to side he watched the patterns made by the light and shade on the under-side of the leaf until his eyes became heavier and heavier. He hummed gently to himself and—

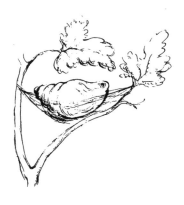

—soon he fell into a deep sleep. He no longer heard the comings and goings in the garden. He did not see Mr. Sun pass through the garden or Queen Moon rise in the evening. He did not feel the rain fall on the leaves or see the grass growing around him. He slept and he slept and he slept.

In his sleep he travelled. He was able to see all of the garden as if he was standing high above it; his legs no longer felt tired and he dreamt that he had grown big beautiful arms painted the colour of some of the brightest flowers in the garden and he felt as light as air. For the first time, as he started to wake up he did not feel cross or tired. He felt as if today was going to bring something new and special, as if something magical was going to happen.

Squat with arms to the sides. Gently flap arms up and down.

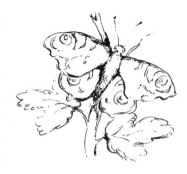

He opened his eyes and found that he was covered in morning dew. He shivered and shook himself. To his surprise he started to lift up into the air. He shook himself again and tried to stretch, expecting his head and body to feel heavy. As he stretched, two large and two smaller beautiful wings unfurled from where his legs used to be. Shaking off the last of the morning dew, he spread his wings and flew out into the sunlight. Below him he could see Dizzy preening herself in preparation for a new day. For a moment he flew between her and Mr. Sun, casting a shadow.

Spread the arms, slowly stand up and run around, slowly flapping arms up and down.
Pause as if resting on leaf for 5 seconds.
Run again.
Pause.
Repeat a few times.

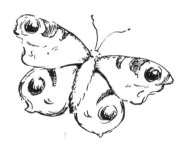

'Oh Mr. Sun, please don't go away so soon', Dizzy said, as she started to uncurl her petals to greet another new day.

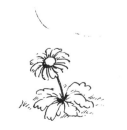

The story can be extended and used with with music.

A number of years ago, I invited Michael Lazarev* to write some music to accompany exercises that I had devised as part of a developmental movement programme for use in schools. When he saw the programme, he said that he had already written a set of songs involving similar characters – his 'zoo programme'. He arranged for the words of his songs to be translated into English and I arranged for two English singers to go to Moscow to record his songs for English-speaking children under his direction. I wrote a small booklet with suggested activities to accompany the songs, with illustrations by Sharon Lewis. The result of our joint efforts was *Wings of Childhood*, a collection of songs on CD written to inspire movement and development in young children from 3–7 years of age.

The song collection can simply be enjoyed as a delightful collection of songs for children to sing along with their parents. It can also be used as the basis for a music and movement programme, encouraging children to act out through movement the 'characters' in the songs. The animal characters have been specially selected based on developmental principles of movement. Practice of these early stages of movement can help prepare children for more advanced skills later on.

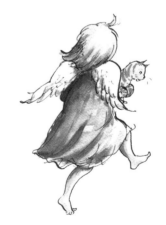

The songs have been recorded using bass and soprano voices to provide as wide a range as possible of sound frequencies involving language. (Remember that father's voice is just as important as mother's voice in developing language.) Children should be encouraged to sing along with the songs because it is use of the child's own voice which provides feedback vital to the development of

---

* Dr Michael Lazarev is a professor of medicine and head of the Children's Rehabilitatory Medicine centre in Moscow. He is author of SONATAL (Sound and Birth). Further information about the SONATAL programme can be found at www.sonatal.ru

Further information about The Institute for Neuro-Physiological Psychology (INPP) can be found at www.inpp.org.uk

language. The second part of the CD contains a charming medley of piano improvisations on the songs, to which children and their parents can add their own words and movements. This is, of course, an activity for fathers as well as mothers.

Examples of two of the songs from *Wings of Childhood* can be found below. You will see that 'The Caterpillar' and 'The Butterfly' provide a natural musical sequel to the story above.

Caterpillar

Words by Michael Lazarev

In the garden, when I stroll,
Many cater-pillars crawl.
Lady with a tummy,
Caterpillar's Mummy.
Near, by running water,
Is caterpillar's daughter.
Caterpillar, Caterpillar
Green leaves' royal princess.
Caterpillar, caterpillar
Garden's fairy tale.
Caterpillar, caterpillar
Delicately minces,
Caterpillar, caterpillar
Wiggling its fat tail.

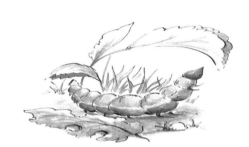

Exercise

Devised by Sally Goddard Blythe

Lie on the tummy, forehead resting on the floor.
Slowly tilt the head up until the back of the head is level with the body.
Pause.
Slowly lower the head down to the ground. Repeat the movement a few times.
When the rhythm of the song starts to change,
(caterpillar, caterpillar, etc), slowly wriggle across the floor in time with the music.

Butterflies

Words by Michael Lazarev

With wings of the butterflies
Fields are a-glitter; in summer
The beautiful butterflies flitter.
From flower to flower
They merrily fly
Winking with a wing's colourful eye.
They hide their bright wings
From the winter-time freeze.
They dream of the summer
And cry for warm breeze.
They wish for the snow to be gone very soon
And the meadows will be covered with flowers in bloom.

Exercise

Stand with arms outstretched.
Wave the arms up and down
like butterfly wings.
On tip-toe,
gently run around the room,
waving the arms,
pausing as if to rest on a flower for a moment
and then, flying on.

In a nutshell

- Children's movement development mirrors stages of evolution.
- See the photographs in Chapter 1 for the sequence of movement development in the first year of life.
- Practice of these movements helps to integrate centres involved in movement control and posture. This can be done through games, stories, songs and activities.
- The story and excerpts from the music CD *Wings of Childhood* provide a 'starter pack' of ideas and ways in which parents can encourage movements, beginning with movements lying on the

floor ('Caterpillar' and 'Tortoise' for example) to crawling ('The bear'), squatting and strutting ('The Peacock') to walking and running ('The deer' and 'Butterflies').

• *Wings of Childhood* can be ordered from www.inpp.org.uk/ publications.

CHAPTER 7

Getting Ready for School

Developmental 'readiness'

The age at which a child becomes ready to read can vary by as much as three years. Some children are eager and ready to start reading by age four, while others can be at least six before the nervous system is ready to support and coordinate all the physical skills needed to facilitate reading. In my experience, many reading problems are the result of either imposing reading expectations on a child who is developmentally not ready, lack of appropriate stimulation in terms of conversation and access to books and stories at home, or failure to recognize specific problems with vision, auditory processing, motor skills or delayed speech. Any one of these problems can interfere with reading, writing, comprehension, numeracy, spelling and social skills later on if they are not recognized.

One of the secrets of success with any type of learning is developmental readiness for the task ahead and ensuring that children are equipped with the necessary tools – in terms of balance, coordination, control of eye movements, hand-eye coordination and listening skills. This is why physical development through the pre-school years is so important for preparing the child to meet the demands of school. The control of eye movements needed to follow a line of letters and words on paper does not develop by itself. Rather, it operates from the platform provided by secure posture and balance. If either posture or balance is unstable, the eye movements needed for reading can be erratic, jumping further along the line when reading, missing out letters and words or even jumping to the line above or the line below. Poor control of eye movements can have the effect of 'scrambling' the information received by the brain from the visual system, with the result that letters on the page are perceived as a jumble of meaningless symbols rather than a sequential flow of coherent information. This has nothing to do with intelligence.

In order to write easily and fluently it is necessary to have not only adequate control of eye movements but cooperation between vision and control of the arm and hand. This is known as visual-motor integration (VMI), and is also closely linked to maturity in the control of posture and balance. In other words, reading and writing begin with control of the *body*.

While practice at reading, writing and fine motor skills is important to familiarize a child with letter shapes, forms and sounds and to *improve* performance, if a child continues to struggle with mastering the basics or does not improve with practice, he may need extra time to develop the underlying physical and motor skills which support control of eye movements and visual-motor integration. This can often be done through the process of play, developing each of the sensory systems and integration between them through *active* learning – learning with the body.

What sort of activities help to improve balance?

Activities to stimulate balance

The balance mechanism comprises three semi-circular canals, each of which responds to a different plane of movement:

- The first plane is rotation around a vertical axis. Carousels, spinning boards and rotating playground equipment provide this type of (passive) stimulation but it can also be actively entrained through activities that involve turning in space. Nursery rhymes and games such as 'Ring-a-Ring-a-Roses' (see pp. 74–5) and 'Here we go round the Mulberry Bush' (pp. 85–7) provide active stimulation, as do traditional country dances and circle dancing.
- The second is rotation or movement through a horizontal axis. This involves forwards and backwards movements such as moving

on a swing, see-saw, rocking horse, rocking chair, turning somersaults and games like 'Row, Row, Row your Boat' (see p. 111).
• The third are tilting movements from side to side. These can be
accomplished by carrying out activities on a wobble board or
surface, which tilts from side to side, space ball etc.

An additional component of the balance mechanism responds specifically to up and down movements: examples of this type of movements include rebound activities such as bouncing on a trampoline,
jumping, and going down a slide.

The balance mechanism is also acutely sensitive to any *alteration*
in speed, or when movement stops and starts (it ceases to react once
movement is steady and constant). Some children have poor control
of static balance (the ability to balance while sitting or standing still)
or in adjusting when movement slows down or stops. These are the
children who tend to be 'on the go' all the time, finding it difficult to
sit still and pay attention. This is because they need to be in motion
to be in control of their body. The most advanced level of movement
control is actually the ability to stay totally still,[1] and when balance
is insecure increased movement or speed of movement is used to
compensate.

For example, can you remember what it was like learning to
ride a bicycle? Once you started moving at a reasonable pace – if
a grown-up ran alongside you pushing the bicycle to get it going
– control of balance improved, but when movement slowed down
or you stopped, the degree of wobble increased and an additional
foot was needed for support. In other words, speed compensates
for instability. This is why activities such as the one suggested in
the story in the previous chapter carried out by 'Wenna the Wood
Louse' are useful in improving adaptation when movement stops
and starts. First, she slowly turns round once and then stops and
closes her eyes. The pause is important to allow the fluid in the
inner ear to settle down before she slowly turns in the opposite
direction. This movement can also be carried out on hands and
knees or standing up.

Activities for touch

There are two types of touch receptor: defensive and discriminatory. The first acts as a protective mechanism from potentially harmful tactile stimuli by attempting to block sensation from travelling further into the nervous system; the second allows information received through touch to enter deeper into the nervous system to be processed and integrated with information received from other senses. Children can be over-sensitive (hyper-sensitive) or under-sensitive (hypo-sensitive) to touch sensations, or in some cases have a combination of both. This can manifest itself in many different ways: from dislike of being hugged to being seemingly unaware of bumping into objects or people; from either avoiding touching to having a compulsive need to touch or an abnormally low or high tolerance of pain. The sense of touch is important for forming an internal 'map' of where parts of the body are in space and knowing where the inner self meets the external environment. Issues related to touch sensitivity are sometimes a feature of disorders linked to body dysmorphia (distorted sense of body image).

Touch is the earliest of the sensory systems to develop, showing signs of response as early as five-and-a-half to seven weeks after conception. In the early months of life a child's experience of being touched should be a gentle one and there are various ways in which parent and infant can enjoy communicating through touch. Feeding, bath and changing times are obvious ones. Infant massage is another.[2]

As children get older, the sense of touch becomes more robust, and can be further developed through movement and activity. If a baby lies on the floor on his tummy, as he learns to support his weight on his hands and later forearms, the palms of the hand are stimulated and the fingers gradually learn to uncurl in response to touch. Kicking the legs, with the feet occasionally coming into contact with the floor, helps a baby to know where his body begins and ends; and when he burrows his toes into the ground to push off to crawl, the gripping reflex in the feet is gradually transformed. Gentle tickling and clapping games such as 'Round and Round the Garden' (see p. 83), 'Pat-a cake, Pat-a-cake, Baker's Man' (see p. 82) and in the older child, rough and tumble play, all help to develop the balance between adequate defence against unwanted stimuli, discrimination of useful stimuli and development of more refined movements.

In early development, movements of the whole hand precede the development of fine finger movements. This is why some of the aforementioned hand games are useful because a child must learn to open and close the *whole* hand at will *before* he can learn to control the individual fingers movements needed to hold and manipulate a writing instrument. When voluntary control of alternately opening and closing the whole hand has been mastered, games which encourage the use of a pincer grip and individual finger movements can be used. Activities which can develop use of the whole hand in children over three are sand play, modelling with materials such as playdough and plasticine, playing with 'potty putty', use of a sponge and squeezy toys in the bath, and helping Mum make pastry, however messy the process!

In the slightly older child, playing a musical instrument is an excellent way of developing hand and finger movements, but equally games such 'Spillikins', 'Jenga' and 'Jacks' are good for developing a pincer grip, independent use of the fingers and hand-eye coordination. The most important factor in any of these activities is that they should be *fun* and that the child should be able to *succeed* at what he is trying to do. If the task is made too difficult, a child will usually give up. Repeated failure tends to be demotivating, while success usually leads to perseverance.

More general rough and tumble play is also important because it not only encourages integrated functioning of the different sensory systems but also recruits and exercises many brain areas and abilities from the brainstem at the base of the brain right up to the somatosensory cortex at the top, promoting general physical fitness and helping to teach regulation of strength and self-control within social settings. It also improves general proprioceptive awareness – the information derived from feedback received from the muscles, tendons and joints concerning body position in space. Proprioceptive awareness is important for developing an internal

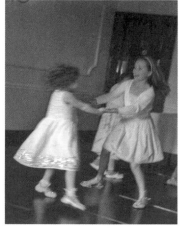

Figure 7.1 Children at play

bodymap, knowing where you are in space and how much strength and movement is needed to carry out physical tasks successfully.

The combination of physical contact and free play arising in rough and tumble play also affect the body's neurochemistry, possibly by increasing brain opioids that create feelings of social strength similar to the effects of the hormone oxytocin, which is known to act as a powerful chemical agent in the forming of social bonds, particularly between mother and child in the first days after birth. Through the exercise of these circuits, rough and tumble play affects the highest regions of the brain (the cortex) because it involves regulation, problem solving, seeking and innovative behaviour in cooperation with the motor system. Jaak Panksepp[3] described how during play, 'animals are especially prone to behave in flexible and creative ways' and that in addition to the effects on muscular development, this type of play probably also 'promotes the generation of new ideas and has a major adaptive function in generating a powerful positive emotional state'.

Free play is different from formal learning because it seems to lack any clear goal other than the process of play itself. Rough and tumble play often involves movements borrowed from other behaviours such as chasing, fleeing, play-fighting, stalking etc. This type of play engages in dangerous pursuits within a relatively safe setting – a practice ground for the regulation of survival behaviours, which will need to be adapted to social settings later on.

In an earlier book I wrote:

> Rough and tumble play occurs most intensely in early life when the brain is developing and neural connections are being formed. It is usually pleasurable and uses considerable energy; it is also social. Social play (other than formal games such as board games) usually involves practice of movement, agility and skill in space, or control of strength. Animals will chase, catch and tussle with each other. Birds will play as a flock, diving from the branches of trees to breakfast from a shrub of berries in the autumn, engaged in an elaborate race to see who can get there first, collect their booty and get out of the way before the next one arrives. Most of all, play should be **fun** and one of the hallmarks of play circuitry in action, is laughter. The importance of laughter for life is greatly under-estimated in the modern world especially in the upbringing and education of children.[4]

Activities to develop auditory skills

Hearing and listening are not identical processes. Hearing describes the ability of the ear to sense sounds, but listening requires more conscious effort and attention to focus on specific sounds, occlude others, interpret the sounds and assign meaning to them.

As discussed in earlier chapters, the unborn child is able hear from as early as 24 weeks after conception and, according to Lazarev, a child can become an attentive listener even before birth if the mother starts a dialogue with her unborn child. Many factors can interfere with a child's ability to listen from hearing impairment, a history of frequent ear, nose or throat infections in the early years, abusive, neglectful or disengaged parents, living in an environment where there is constant background noise, auditory hypersensitivity or problems with attention.* These are just a few of the possible contributory factors. More important is what parents can do to avoid problems developing, or to help a child overcome them.

Earlier chapters have covered many ideas for developing auditory skills. Key elements are: talking-listening-responding to your infant; being responsive when he wants to engage with you; talking to your child while you share daily activities; singing to your child; singing with your child; telling stories and *reading* to your child *every* day; teaching your child the importance of taking turns in conversation and not interrupting. Chapters 3–5 contain ideas for musical games to play and stories to read your child.

---

* Every day, environmental distractors increase in number. From the bleeping of electronic message alerts, computers being turned on, electronic timers reminding us when it is time to do something, TV or radio on at home, or background music in public places, the modern world interrupts children's attempts to focus on one task every few seconds. Children are being schooled from birth to divert attention to novel stimuli every few seconds – daily lessons in attention deficit.

 Too many stimuli competing for attention at one time also increase stress and can reduce efficiency in processing information.

 If there is too much competing background noise it becomes difficult not only to focus on one source of sound but to hear a single voice above the general background noise level.

We have done all the things suggested, but our child still does not seem to be 'ready' for school

If your child has reached the statutory age for formal education but does not seem to be responding to teaching or is having problems fitting in socially, the first step is to ask:

1 What?
2 Why?

1 In **what** areas is your child experiencing difficulty?
   - Is the child's behavior different at home and at school?
   - In what situations is he struggling?
   - Was he born during the summer months? Children born in June, July and August are biologically 9–12 months younger than their peers throughout their school career. This can be particularly important in the early years if they are not ready in terms of their physical skills at the time of school entry. If they fall behind at this time in the mastery of basic skills, it can be much harder to catch up later on. These children can trail behind their classmates not because they lack ability but because they are continuously playing 'catch-up'.

2 **Why** is he struggling?
   There can be many reasons why a child struggles in the first year at school. A few areas which might indicate the need for further investigation are listed below but please note that generally a *cluster* of symptoms need to be present.

Indications of neuro-motor immaturity in the school-aged child

- Does he have problems sitting still?
- Does he tend to slump down on to the desk when writing?
- Does he have an awkward pencil grip, which he reverts to even when shown how to hold it correctly?
- Does he have difficulty doing up buttons, or putting clothes on the right way round?
- Does he have difficulty using a knife and fork correctly?

- Does he have difficulty catching a ball?
- Does he appear to be significantly more awkward than other children of the same age in the playground or at P.E?
- When using his hands for a task do you see reciprocal mouth movements or vice-versa?
- Does he complain the words and letters 'move' on the page?
- Is there a marked discrepancy between his progress in reading and writing?
- If asked to copy simple shapes such as a circle, square and X, is he able to copy the shapes correctly?
- Can he stand on one leg without falling over or putting the other foot on the floor: for six seconds at age four, and eight seconds at age five?
- Can he draw a circle in the air in both a clockwise and anti-clockwise direction?

If a *cluster* of problems in the above checklist continue to affect your child above the age of six, it is possible that immature neuro-motor skills underlie some of his presenting difficulties. Neuro-motor skills can be improved with the use of specific therapeutic programmes such as Sensory Integration Therapy (SI) which can be prescribed by a trained Occupational Therapist, or either of the INPP programmes.

INPP offers two types of neuro-motor programme:

1   A general programme of developmental movements designed to be used in schools with a whole class of children.[5] Exercises are carried out every day under teacher supervision for one academic year. A short battery of developmental tests is included for teachers to assess children's progress at the beginning and the end of the year.

2   An individual programme tailored to the child's specific needs. This programme is carried out at home for five to ten minutes per day under parental supervision following a thorough neuro-motor assessment. The child's progress is reassessed at two-monthly intervals and the developmental movement programme is adjusted accordingly. The duration of the programme is approximately one year.[6]

What is neuro-motor immaturity?

INPP uses the term neuro-motor immaturity to describe the continued presence of a cluster of abnormal primitive and postural reflexes in a child above three-and-a-half years of age. Immature reflexes affect postural abilities and dependent motor skills, and can undermine motor performance and resulting skills in the older child. Delay in general motor milestones such as age of sitting, crawling and walking in the first year of life may be indicative of immature development in the supporting reflex system. Both general motor milestones in the first years of life and abnormal primitive and postural reflexes in the older child provide indications of neuro-motor maturity.

Identification of possible signs of delay in the first years is important to enable parents and teachers to:

- define or eliminate the possibility of the disorder causing developmental concerns (e.g. mental retardation, cerebral palsy, autism, hearing impairment, communication disorders).
- investigate the underlying causes of the disorder (e.g. metabolic or genetic disorder, injury due to oxygen deprivation (anoxic) or toxic exposure (e.g. drugs used by the mother during pregnancy, lead exposure etc.);
- assess for the presence of associated disorders;
- direct intervention services and follow up needs;
- provide appropriate counsel to the child's family regarding the implications of the diagnosis.[7]

What are the risk factors for neuro-motor immaturity linked to developmental delay?

Risk factors for developmental problems may be twofold:

- Genetic
- Environmental

Examples of genetic factors include being born with a genetic or chromosomal abnormality. Down's syndrome is one example of a disorder that causes developmental delay as a result of an extra, abnormal chromosome.

Environmental risks are numerous, ranging from exposure to harmful agents either before or after birth, which can have a profound effect upon development, to minor events, or the cumulative impact of several minor events, which have milder and more subtle consequences in the longer term.

Agents known to have an adverse effect on the embryo and foetus are called 'teratogens' and include exposure to toxins such as prescription and non-prescription drugs at key stages in pregnancy or infections that are passed directly from a mother to baby during pregnancy such as rubella or syphilis.

Poor maternal nutrition, and exposure to alcohol and smoking can all affect the foetus in different ways, depending on the time in pregnancy when exposure occurred, quantity and duration of exposure. The unborn child is most vulnerable to damage from external agents in the first eight to twelve weeks after conception. This is the time when the major organs are being formed and is before the placental barrier has been established. The placenta acts rather like a filter which provides protection to the developing baby from most harmful substances, but the foetus can be affected at any time during pregnancy.

Additional environmental risk factors include a child's life experiences. Premature birth for example places children at greater potential risk, as does being conceived as by in vitro fertilization (IVF),*

---

* Risk factors associated with IVF start with the reason(s) for failure to conceive. This may be to do with the quality of sperm, egg, problems in the female reproductive tract or compatibility issues between father and mother; the process of selection in IVF is not nearly as rigorous as natural selection where millions of sperm will be wasted in favour of one that is strong enough to swim to the egg, to penetrate the ovum and for the mother's body not to reject the zygote as a foreign invading body; hormones often need to be prescribed to the mother before IVF to stimulate egg release and after implantation to secure the pregnancy. It has been suggested that exposure to elevated levels of certain hormones in the womb can have subtle effects on brain development. Although the practice of implanting several embryos is now being phased out, many IVF pregnancies start off as twin pregnancies. Sometimes one twin is miscarried, or, if both survive, there is an increased risk of premature birth and the need for obstetric intervention at birth. Children born prematurely are at increased risk of later health and learning problems. Children born as a result of IVF have poor nutrition, maternal depression, severe poverty, lack of care, neglect, or abuse – although there is no certain causation between these potential risk factors and the emergence of later difficulties. Risk factors have a cumulative impact upon development. As the number of risk factors increases, a child is put at greater risk of problems associated with developmental delay.[8]

How is a developmental delay identified?

Developmental delay is identified firstly through screening, and secondly, through evaluation.

1 Screening

Developmental screening tests provide a quick and general measurement of skills in relation to chronological age although they may also include developmental history. Screening tests should not be used as the basis for a diagnosis, but can be useful as an indicator for further developmental evaluation.

2 Evaluation

Evaluation involves in-depth assessment of a child's skills in one or several areas and should be administered by a highly trained professional. In the United Kingdom, access to professionals qualified in the assessment of developmental problems is generally made through referral by the child's general practitioner. If problems emerge within the educational environment, referral is generally made by a professional such as an educational psychologist.

---

therefore often been exposed to a *sequence* of risk factors before they are born. This is not to say that children born as a result of IVF will develop problems, but the long-term consequences on a child's development of IVF are not yet well documented. In a survey of 80 children seen at INPP in Chester between December 2008 and December 2009 because they had some sort of learning or behavioural problem, ten percent had been conceived as a result of IVF. Ten years ago this figure was nil.

Evaluation tests are used to create a profile of a child's strengths and weaknesses in all developmental areas. The results of a developmental evaluation are used to determine if the child is in need of treatment by early intervention services.

Early intervention services

Early intervention services include a variety of different resources and programmes that provide specific intervention for the child and support to families. These include:

- Health visitors
- Audiology or hearing services
- Orthoptic services – the evaluation and nonsurgical treatment of visual disorders caused by imbalance of the eye muscles, such as strabismus (squint)
- Child and Adolescent Mental Health Service (CAMHS)
- Educational programmes
- Occupational therapy
- Physical therapy
- Psychological services
- Speech/Language
- Access to assistive technology

Early identification and intervention are important to help a child advance in all areas of development. Delay in one area can affect other developmental areas. For example, a child with visual impairment may have coordination difficulties, poor spatial skills, and anxiety in new situations; hearing problems can affect the development of speech and language, reading and spelling, and behaviour. Immature motor skills can affect posture, coordination, control of eye movements, non-verbal language and behaviour. It is therefore vital that a child's underlying problems are identified and intervention happens as early as possible. If you have any concerns about your child's physical development prior to starting school, discuss these with your Health Visitor or GP.

Other specific areas that might underlie failure to progress at school include hearing or listening problems, visual impairment and visual-perceptual problems.

Indicators of auditory problems

There are two types of hearing loss: **sensori-neural** and **conductive**.

Sensori-neural hearing loss is a type of hearing loss which results from either damage to the vestibulo-cochlear nerve (the nerve which conducts vibrations from the ear to the brain) or the inner ear, or central processing centres of the brain. Sensori-neural hearing loss is permanent. The degree of sensori-neural hearing loss can be mild, moderate, severe, or profound. Sometimes the loss is progressive (hearing gradually becomes poorer) and sometimes unilateral (one ear only).

Conductive hearing loss describes hearing impairment which is due to an interference in the transmission of sound to the inner ear before it reaches the cochlea (the organ of hearing). The most common cause of conductive hearing loss in infants and children is an infection of the middle ear (Otitis Media). This is usually treated with antibiotics, or in persistent or severe cases, with surgery. Hearing can usually be restored following treatment but if there have been frequent bouts of intermittent hearing loss in the first three years of life, (during the time a child 'tunes in' to the sounds of the mother tongue), problems with the *processing* of auditory information can persist even after the primary hearing impairment has been resolved.

High risk factors for sensori-neural hearing loss (SNHL)

- Family history of sensori-neural hearing loss
- History of infection during pregnancy with toxoplasmosis, rubella, cytomegalovirus, herpes, syphilis
- Ear or other cranio-facial abnormalities
- Hyperbilirubinaemia at levels requiring exchange transfusion
- Birth weight of less than 1500g
- Bacterial meningitis
- Low Apgar scores at each assessment

- Respiratory distress (e.g. meconium aspiration)
- Physical features associated with a syndrome known to include SNHL, e.g. Down's Syndrome, Williams's Syndrome
- Recurrent or persistent Otitis Media for at least 3 months
- Childhood infections associated with SNHL, e.g. meningitis, mumps or measles
- Ototoxic medication (e.g. gentamicin) administered for more than five days

Risk factors and indicators for auditory processing problems

- Delay in speech or language development
- History of failed hearing tests
- History of repeated ear, nose, throat or chest infections in the first three years of life
- Mouth breather/snores at night
- Chronic and persistent rhinitis
- History of surgery for removal of tonsils or adenoids, or insertion of grommets

Indicators of hearing or auditory processing difficulties

- Does not respond when spoken to the first time or when out of sight
- Tends to shout
- Speech indistinct
- Mishears words or instructions
- Mispronunciation of specific sounds
- Need for frequent repetition when given instructions
- Slow to respond to spoken questions of information
- Difficulty coping with background noise
- Seemingly unaware of people and objects outside the range of peripheral vision
- History of difficulty chewing or swallowing 'chunky' food
- Cannot pronounce similar sounds correctly eg. *m* and *n*; *b* and *p*; *p* and *d*; *f* and *th*; *sh* and *ch*; *g* and *x*.

- Has the TV on loud
- Dislike of certain sounds which do not bother other people

If a number of the above factors are applicable and have not responded to previous intervention, it is possible that auditory factors might be affecting progress in other areas, including education. If hearing problems of any kind are suspected these should first be checked out with a thorough hearing assessment. A hearing test and other tests for auditory functioning can be arranged through your doctor.

If the medical assessments of hearing are normal, but your child still has a *cluster* of the behavioural signs listed under 'indicators' above, there are various methods of sound therapy, which can help to improve *listening* skills. These therapies involve listening to specially filtered music that can help to improve auditory discrimination (the ability to differentiate between similar sounds such *b* and *d*, *p* and *b*, *t* and *d*, *sh* and *ch*, etc.), auditory delay (slower than normal at processing the sounds of speech) and hypersensitivity to specific sounds.

Johansen Individualized Auditory Stimulation (JIAST) is one such programme. Following a thorough auditory assessment, a special CD is made of frequency-specific music, which has been customized to the child's individual hearing curve. The child listens to the CD for ten minutes a day and is reassessed at intervals for a period of nine to twelve months. New CDs are made at follow-up visits following auditory re-assessment. This programme is suitable for children from about four years of age and upwards, although hearing assessments may need to be adjusted according to the age and attention span of the child.

Other methods of Sound Therapy include the Tomatis Method, the Listening Fitness Programme (LiFT), Auditory Integrative Training (AIT), The Listening Programme (TLP) and Musica Medica. The most suitable method of sound therapy depends on the presenting symptoms and underlying causes of the child's difficulty and should be selected on the basis of individual assessment and individual needs.

Before the mid 1980s, at the time of school entry every child was assessed by a school doctor who carried out simple tests to assess balance, coordination, hearing and vision. These tests are no longer carried out as a matter of routine, with the result that some children with coordination, hearing and visual problems slip through the net on entering the school system, and lack the basic physical equipment needed to support academic learning.

I regularly see children in my practice who have come to me because they have problems with reading and writing but who, on assessment of basic eye movements, are suspected of having a mild degree of long sightedness. Referral to an optometrist and the use of just a low-level glasses prescription for close work can make all the difference, as it would for anyone in middle age when they start to develop long sight and struggle to thread a needle or read the newspaper. I have also noticed an increase in this problem in younger children and suspect it is connected with increased use of electronic devices including computers in the early years, which require children to maintain focus at a distance slightly further than a normal reading distance. Whatever the cause, it is essential that a child should have adequate vision, visual skills and visual perception in order to succeed in the classroom.

Indicators of visual processing problems (general)

- Eyes not lined up correctly, i.e. one eye drifts or aims in a different direction from the other
- Consistently turns or tilts head to see
- Head is frequently tilted to one side
- Closing or covering of one eye
- Excessive blinking or squinting
- Avoids close work
- Poor handwriting
- Poor hand-eye coordination
- Problems moving in space, frequently bumps into things or drops things
- Clumsiness in playground or at home
- Difficulty catching or hitting a ball
- Able to read for only short periods of time
- Complains of regular or persistent headaches or eyestrain
- Nausea or dizziness when carrying out close work
- Motion sickness
- Double vision

Indicators at near distance

- Holds the book or object very close or far away
- Closes or covers one eye
- Twists or tilts head to carry out task
- Frequently loses place
- Uses finger or pointer to read
- Rubs eyes during or after short periods of reading
- Reversals when reading (i.e., 'was' for 'saw', 'on' for 'no', etc.)
- Reversals when writing (*b* for *d*, *p* for *q*, etc.)
- Misses out small words
- Transposition of letters and numbers (12 for 21, etc.)
- Omits words or lines when reading
- Complains that letters or text 'move' on the page
- Marked discrepancy between oral and written work

Any suspected problems with vision should be investigated by an optometrist. Many visual problems arise purely from eyesight and these can easily be remedied with corrective lenses. Problems with visual *processing* (how the brain interprets information from the eyes) can also be related to oculo-**motor** dysfunction.

Oculo-motor problems (control of eye *movements*) can be linked to specific ocular problems such as strabismus (cross eyed) which may need either specific visual training or in the last resort, surgical intervention, or they may stem from more general neuro-motor immaturity, which in many cases will respond to a specific motor training programme.

Some children have difficulty with light contrast, which affects their ability to see black print on white paper and can affect other areas of visual processing such as depth perception and pattern recognition. Originally described by Dr Helen Irlen as Irlen Syndrome or Scotopic Sensitivity Syndrome (SSS), this syndrome can be diagnosed by a trained Irlen practitioner or identified by specialist optometrists. The use of coloured overlays or prescribed tinted lenses can help to overcome this problem in the short term in some cases.

Individual differences in rates of development

Although there are general timelines at which children are expected to reach major developmental milestones such as sitting, crawling, walking and talking, there can be considerable individual variation in rates of development. Rudolf Steiner observed that reading readiness naturally occurs at the about the same time as a child starts to shed his first milk teeth, usually between six and six-and-a-half. This is the same age that children *start* formal school in many other European countries and in the United States. In other words, other educational systems allow children an extended period of time in the early years to develop the range of physical skills needed to support academic learning. Children in the United Kingdom start school at rising five years of age and are expected to start formal instruction in reading, writing and numeracy and to reach targets at least one year earlier than their European counterparts. In Finland, children do not begin formal instruction in reading until they are seven. Comparative studies suggest that this does not disadvantage them.

If your child seems to be lagging behind in some of the physical skills needed to support learning, the general advice is to provide them with as much opportunity as possible to enjoy and develop physical skills as a normal part of daily life.

Boys and girls also differ in their rates of development:

Males, often viewed as the physically stronger sex are actually more vulnerable in the early years than females, suffering a significantly higher rate of spontaneous abortion, premature birth, infant mortality, a range of illnesses in the early years including ear, nose and throat infections, and a tendency to be fussier and more irritable in infancy. They are also more likely to suffer from developmental disorders including autism, attention deficit disorder and dyslexia.

Greater susceptibility to this range of problems is thought to result from a combination of larger brain size and slower rate of maturation before birth, the presence of only one X chromosome and exposure to higher levels of pre-natal testosterone. Testosterone depresses the functioning of the immune system.[9]

While girls appear to have advantages in the early years, the scales start to even out at puberty, when girls' growth and maturation slows down about two years earlier than that of boys. By the mid-twenties, many earlier biological developmental differences in learning outcomes level off – provided that both sexes have enjoyed equal opportunity to develop in ways supportive to gender specific learning needs. Despite many recognized behavioural differences between the sexes, differences in the architecture of the brain are surprisingly small and are thought to result largely from pre-natal exposure to different hormones, particularly testosterone. The effects of small differences in hormonal environment increase with time and at different stages of development resulting in divergence in how the brains of boys and girls function.

The most profound difference between girls and boys is in the **sequence of development** of the various brain regions. A study published in 2007 demonstrated that there is **no overlap in the trajectories of brain development** in girls and boys,[10] showing that they develop different skills at different times and in different ways. This finding is supported by other studies which investigated specific skills in young children, including one which examined two-year-olds building bridges out of blocks. Even at age two, boys were about three times more likely than girls to be able to build a bridge out of blocks,[11] while another study found that three-and-a-half-year-old girls were better at interpreting facial expressions than five-year-old boys.[12] In other words, maturation alone is not the whole story.

Despite general differences, of course, there can be considerable individual variation in relation to specific criteria. These natural differences are reinforced by nurture, cultural expectations and experience. While genes and hormones set the scene, experience can amplify or diminish differences. This raises the question of how education can foster and accommodate these different rates of maturation, needs and learning styles to bring out the best in both boys and girls.

Some of the acknowledged differences between boys and girls

- Boys grow more quickly than girls from early on in gestation and male cells have a higher metabolic rate, making them potentially more vulnerable to damage at stages of rapid proliferation.

- Boys have a slower rate of maturation in the respiratory and immune systems before birth, making them more susceptible to illnesses in the early years.
- Boys' brains are larger than female brains (about nine percent larger), but girls mature at a physiologically faster rate up to puberty.
- More boys than girls suffer foetal distress during the birth process and have lower Apgar scores at birth, making them more vulnerable to damage.
- Newborn boys secrete more stress hormone in response to a surprise stimulus than girls, making them more reactive to certain stimuli.
- Girls are ahead of boys in the early aspects of expressive language including use of gesture and first words (about one month earlier), vocabulary growth (about two months earlier in toddler-hood) and about 15 per cent more verbally fluent than boys at four to five years of age. There is no difference in receptive language at five years of age.[13]
- Boys are generally better at visuo-spatial tasks, while girls are ahead in verbal skills.
- Boys are usually superior in strength and endurance in gross motor skills but slower at developing fine motor skills.
- Boys are physically more active and impulsive, and less likely to calm themselves than girls.

What are the positive aspects of male difference and how can these be nurtured in the educational environment?

In general, the male brain is wired to respond in external, rather than internal, ways. This can leave boys at a disadvantage in a school environment, when teaching focuses on the sedentary development of verbal skills at the expense of more active learning. As early as kindergarten, kinetic, impulsive boys are told to sit down, be quiet, and do their work. Teachers are expected to provide a calm, controlled classroom, but boys tend to learn by doing, and if activity in the classroom is suppressed they need to 'let off steam' in other, physical ways.

Regular physical activity can be introduced easily into the school day. The 'Fit for Learning' programme is one example. Developed by Professor Pat Preedy and Chris Lees at a primary school in the Midlands, 'Fit for Learning' enables teachers to break up learning sessions with physical activities. The sessions are led by teachers and require no preparation, minimum space and resources. Staff have reported significant improvements in children's coordination, behaviour and concentration.[14] These empirical findings mirror standard practice in other cultures such as Japan and Taiwan where twice as many break times are incorporated into the school day in the early years, and educational attainment remains high.

Normal attention span is approximately equivalent to three to five minutes for each year of a child's age. A two-year-old should therefore be able to concentrate on a particular task for up to six minutes, and a child entering kindergarten should be able to concentrate for 15 minutes. The longer a child has to sit still beyond her natural attention span, the greater the amount of fidgeting, vocal activity and general disruption. In Finland, pre-school education pays particular attention to the physical needs of children, incorporating up to two hours of outdoor play into the pre-school day. This enables boys to work out their physical energy while encouraging girls to develop gross motor skills, resulting in a more level playing field when all children begin formal instruction in reading at age seven.

Boys need extra encouragement to develop verbal skills in the early years, because reading ability grows out of spoken language. Language develops through use not just through passive listening. This may partly be why simply watching/listening to the TV or radio – despite the verbal component – has been shown to have a deleterious effect on language development in young children. 'Sounding out' is an important precursor to being able to decode visual symbols phonologically, and sounding out begins with speech, conversation, telling stories and singing. Singing, sometimes erroneously regarded as a 'girl' activity, can help prepare the voice, the eye and the brain for reading and is suited to boys because it involves active learning. As mentioned earlier, cathedral choristers provide examples of how regular singing can enhance every aspect of academic learning.[15]

Physical readiness also plays an important part in a child's ability to sit still, pay attention, hold and control a writing implement and to transfer thoughts via the motor system onto paper. While boys' gross motor skills are generally more robust than those of girls, they tend to struggle for longer to master fine motor skills. Problems with writing can be minimized by separating the mechanics of writing from cognitive processing, teaching penmanship as one skill, and encouraging them to talk about ideas and answers before putting them on to paper.

Rough and tumble play is also important for boys because it allows children to explore in creative ways and to test boundaries of strength and control without aggression. In ancient Greece, athletics and wrestling were important elements of a boy's education, as control of the body was considered essential training for the mind. Wrestling was used to develop control of strength and temper. All healthy young mammals engage in rough and tumble play and there is a correlation between the appearance of this type of activity and maturity in the frontal lobes of the brain – which are involved in creativity, imagination, empathy, planning and self-control.

One reason suggested by leading scientist Jaak Panksepp for the increasing incidence of ADHD amongst children (particularly boys) may be:

> ... the diminishing availability of opportunities for pre-school children to engage in natural self-generated social play. Pre-clinical work indicates that play can facilitate behavioral inhibition in growing animals, while psychostimulants (ritalin for example) reduce playfulness. The idea that intensive social play interventions, throughout early childhood, may alleviate ADHD symptoms remains to be evaluated. As an alternative to the use of play-reducing psychostimulants, society could establish play 'sanctuaries' for at-risk children in order to facilitate frontal lobe maturation and the healthy development of pro-social minds.[16]

These recommendations were confirmed recently by Dr Abigail Norfleet James, author of *Teaching the Male Brain*.[17] Speaking at The International Boys' Schools Coalition (IBSC) conference in central London in January 2010, she said that boys and girls have distinct skills, with boys generally being less verbal, having less acute hearing, slower perceptual speed and being less likely to be able to control their impulses. In contrast, boys generally have better spatial skills, more acute vision, learn best through touch, are more impulsive, more physically active and are 'movement orientated'[18] throughout primary and secondary education.

If boys and girls are to have equality of opportunity in education, then education needs to take these small but significant differences in rates of maturation and learning needs into account from the outset.[19]

What can be done to help boys who struggle at fine motor tasks such as writing?

Writing problems can arise for at least two reasons:

1   Difficulty in controlling the pencil, stemming from problems with motor control, or visual-motor integration difficulties.
2   Difficulty in sequencing ideas and being able to express them using the motor system.

Boys tend to be later at developing the fine motor skills needed for writing. If all concentration must be focused on the *mechanics* of writing it can interfere with the ability to think and write at the same time, hence a discrepancy between oral ability, reading and written performance.

Separating handwriting as a skill (penmanship) from creative writing or copying of content can help to develop the mechanics of writing first. Suggestions as to how this can be done include:

- Encouraging boys to copy the shapes and contours of large letters as a 'drawing' skill in the early years.
- Getting boys to draw and talk about their ideas before writing them down.
- Providing paper with double narrow lines as guidelines for letter formation. Letters must be kept inside the two lines, with the exception of short- tall letters such as *t* and *p*, and tall-tall letters such as *h, d, b, l, k,* etc. which extend above or below the lines.
- Encouraging a boy to 'tell' the story he wants to write first. You can then write the main points down for him, which he then copies out.

Occasionally children with writing problems have retained an infant reflex (ATNR), which interferes with hand-eye coordination. Special exercises designed to inhibit the reflex can improve the mechanical aspects of writing.

Gaps in the system

At the time of writing, despite the many services available to provide support for children with developmental delay and their families, in real terms gaps in the system continue to exist which mean a failure to identify developmental problems at an early age and refer children for appropriate assessment and effective remediation. There is, for example, no automatic crossover between the fields of medicine and education for referring problems which potentially affect both health and education. This means that children with mild neuro-motor immaturity often simply 'slip through the net' because there is no national screening process in place for children at the time of school entry, or to track development of physical skills once they enter formal education.

Whereas in the early 1980s every child was assessed by a school doctor at rising five years of age on basic motor skills, vision and hearing, these routine tests were phased out a few years later. Teachers are not currently qualified to carry out physical developmental tests on children, and educational psychologists focus primarily on measures of cognitive performance, not underlying physical development. INPP's research in schools between 2000 and 2010 suggests that in the absence of medical screening of children in school, there is a need for teachers to be trained in how to screen for signs of developmental delay, so that appropriate referrals or implementation of proven physical programmes can be introduced into schools.

Until such changes are implemented, in my experience the identification of children's needs remains something of a lottery, with the onus falling on parents to be aware of potential problems, employ preventive measures as far as possible and to seek out relevant help when needed. As with any lottery, there are a few winners and many losers. There is much work still to be done in ensuring that as far as possible all children begin their formal education from a level playing field. Developmental readiness is one starting point for this.

Summary

Human beings have evolved in a context in which the survival of each individual demands continuous adaptation. The adult human brain is the product not only of the genes and heritable characteristics it was born with, but also many years of *interaction* with the physical world. It is the combination of nature *with* nurture, brain *and* body in the milieu of loving and supportive relationships, which make an individual what she is.

In a translated version of writings from Hippocrates dated from 400 BC Hippocrates said that,

> It ought to be known that the source of pleasure, merriment, laughter and amusement, as of our grief, anxiety and tears, is none other than the brain*. It is the brain too, which is the seat of madness and delirium, of the fears and frights which assail us, often by night, but sometimes by day; it is there where lies the cause of insomnia and sleep-walking, of thoughts which will not come, forgotten duties and eccentricities. All such things result from an unhealthy condition of the brain.[20]

While the human brain is now known to be the seat of all conscious thoughts, feelings and imaginings, stored inside this extraordinary blob of matter at birth is the entire evolutionary history of the individual, waiting to unfold its potential. But it cannot do so without the body. It is the body which supports, protects, sustains and nourishes the brain through interaction with its environment. For optimum mental as well as physical health, performance and well-being there needs to be *congruence* in the relationship between the brain and the body. This develops in the context of *relationships* – physical, social and emotional. The human mind (psyche) with all its possibilities is the product of these continuously adapting relationships.

All living things are a combination of matter and energy. Matter describes the physical material of the universe, and energy the capacity

---

* The use of the word brain in this translation is sometimes disputed as at the time it was not known what the brain does. It is more likely that the word 'psyche' applied, which meant soul, spirit, breath and life.

to act upon it in some way. *Quality* of life emerges as a result of the complex interaction between the parts that make up an individual and her environment. As mankind develops ever more complex forms of technology, whose main aim is to reduce the amount of physical or mental energy required by a task, there is a risk that the very physical processes that made it possible for the human brain to contrive and devise such tools, start to atrophy in future generations – unless they receive sufficient stimulus in the form of interaction and experience in the physical world. This is especially important in childhood, as the interaction of sensory and motor experience results in modification of associative functioning in the brain. 'Whenever brain cells are connected in new ways, there comes into existence a physical basis for a new idea in the world of thought.[21] In every idea there is a physical, motor element; and an idea of any concrete thing contains the germ of motor action. In other words, thought is an internalized simulation of motor action. All thought contains a motor element; even simply imagining a static object involves a simulated visual process to 'see' the object in the mind's eye. This is what Berthoz[22] meant when he described thought as being an internalized form of action.

As mankind has become more successful at controlling the environment, the pace of cultural change has increasingly outstripped the slower process of biological change. In the modern world we are in danger of ignoring the fact that every child starts from the same biological beginnings as her ancestors and needs time and opportunity to experience the same biological development stages as her forebears, irrespective of social and cultural change. Traditional games, activities and child-rearing practices of previous generations still have a role in providing a vital link between biological development and culture.

But physical interaction is not the only process that has made us what we are. All mammals and primates share a need for social engagement, social contact and the comfort provided by a primary source of love throughout the years of childhood and adolescence. This was graphically illustrated by experiments which Harlow carried out more than fifty years ago on rhesus monkeys, in which infant monkeys were removed from their mothers and given the choice of two inanimate surrogate mothers.

One surrogate mother was made of terrycloth but provided no food. The other surrogate mother was made of wire and had a feeding bottle attached to it containing milk. It was found that the monkeys consistently turned to the cloth mother for comfort, even though it was not able to provide food, and only went to the wire mother for food. They also formed an emotional attachment to the 'soft' mother, clinging to it when they were placed in an unfamiliar room and returning to her at intervals when they felt secure enough to explore an unfamiliar environment. Monkeys who were placed in unfamiliar surroundings without access to the cloth mother froze in fear, cried, cowered or sucked their thumbs, and some searched frantically for the cloth mother in their distress. Monkeys placed in the same situation with the wire mothers exhibited the same behaviour as the monkeys with no mother. Harlow concluded that the need for contact comfort was stronger than the need to explore. A further implication is that young children need comfort and security to have the confidence to physically explore the boundaries of their environment.

The study also found that while there was no difference in weight gain depending on whether the monkey had been raised with a cloth and wire mother or with a wire mother only, the monkeys that only had access to a wire mother had more trouble digesting the milk, and suffered more frequent episodes of diarrhoea. Harlow's interpretation of their behaviour was that a lack of contact comfort was psychologically stressful to young monkeys and resulted in changes in physiological processes and behaviour.[23] His findings, when translated into human behaviour, suggest that feeding by itself is not the most important factor in forming a parent-child bond; the body contact derived from nursing is also significant.*

Parents, followed by carers, teachers, are the primary sculptors of tomorrow's society. Children were designed to be brought up in an atmosphere of love, physical contact and connection with the outside world. While governments, politicians and civil servants may draw

---

*   I am horrified when I occasionally see mothers give a feeding bottle to a young baby barely able to hold the bottle in place by itself, and abandon the baby in a baby seat while she carries on a conversation and completely ignores her child. One thing that Harlow's experiments did teach us is that contact is important for emotional security and bonding. One of the many advantages of breast feeding is that the infant receives physical contact during feeding.

up the plans for social welfare and education, each and every child needs the opportunity to explore the natural world and engage with people around her. While technology has provided modern society with a wonderful array of tools to make life physically easier, technology (including devices designed to make parents' lives easier such as baby seats, electronic baby-sitters and games) should never *replace* a child's experience of discovering the natural world and her place in it through each and every stage of her development.

As parents you cannot make your children into geniuses, but you can release and share the secrets of natural childhood, which enable children to thrive.

In a nutshell

- Developmental readiness is the key to learning success.
- Balance and control of posture provide a stable platform for the coordination needed to achieve well in the classroom.
- Sensory integration takes place as a result of movement and action. Certain activities can help to develop sensory awareness, integration and improved motor control.
- Physical play, including rough and tumble play, provides a practice ground for life.
- Not all children are 'ready' for school at the time of school entry and it is important to identify signs and causes of immaturity to provide effective remediation and support.
- Boys and girls develop different skills at different rates and at different times. Nurturing these differences throughout development can help all children to succeed.
- When you train the body you also train the brain.

Notes

1   N. Rowe: Personal communication, 1996.
2   Society for Infant Massage. www.iaim.org.uk
3   J. Panksepp: *Affective Neuroscience. The Foundations of Human and Animal Emotions.* Oxford University Press, New York 1998.
4   S.A. Goddard Blythe: *What Babies and Children Really Need.* Hawthorn Press, Stroud 2008.

5 S.A. Goddard Blythe: *The INPP Test Battery and Developmental Movement Programme for Use in Schools with Children with Special Educational Needs.* Restricted Publication, INPP Chester, 1996, revised 1997.

6 The INPP Programme. www.inpp.org.uk/parents

7 A.J. Capute, P.J. Accardo: *Developmental Disabilities in Infancy and Childhood.* Paul Brookes Publishing Company, Baltimore 1991.

8 http://www.howkidsdevelop.com/developDevDelay.html

9 J. Durden-Smith, D. de Simone: *Sex and the Brain.* Pan Books Ltd, London 1983.

10 The NIH/NIMH study: 'Sexual dimorphism of brain developmental trajectories during childhood and adolescence.' *NeuroImage.*36/4: 165–73, 2007.

11 J.C. Labarthe: 'Are boys better than girls at building a tower or a bridge at 2 years of age?' *Archives of Diseases of Childhood.* 77: 140–4, 1997.

12 C. Boyatzis, E. Chazan, C.Z. Ting: 'Preschool children's decoding of facial emotions.' *Journal of Genetic Psychology,* 154: 375–82, 1993.

13 L. Eliot: *Pink Brain, Blue Brain. How Small Differences Grow into Troublesome Gaps – and What We Can Do About It.* Hougton Mifflin Harcourt, New York 2009.

14 Knowle C. of E. School. Knowle, Solihull.

15 S.A. Goddard Blythe: *The Well-Balanced Child.* Hawthorn Press, Stroud 2003.

16 J. Panksepp: 'Can play diminish ADHD and facilitate the construction of the social brain?' J Can Acad Child Adolesc Psychiatry. 16/2: 57–66, 2007.

17 James A. Norfleet: *Teaching the Male Brain.* Corwin Press CA, 2007.

18 James A. Norfleet, presentation at The International Boys' Schools Coalition (IBSC) Conference. London, 19 January 2010.

19 S.A. Goddard Blythe: 'Why boys and girls have different needs in the early years.' Montessori International.95: 14–18, 2010.

20 Cited in: G.E.R Lloyd (ed.): *Hippocratic Writings* (translated J. Chadwick). Penguin Classic Paperbacks. London 1983.

21 R.P. Halleck: *The Education of the Nervous System.* The Macmillan Company, New York 1898.

22 A. Berthoz: *The Brain's Sense of Movement.* Harvard University Press, Cambridge 2000.

23 H.F. Harlow: 'The Nature of Love.' Address to the sixty-sixth Annual Convention of the American Psychological Association, Washington, D.C., August 31, 1958.

Resources

1   Movement programmes

The INPP Individual Programme	www.inpp.org.uk/parents
The INPP School Programme	www.inpp.org.uk/training
Toddler Kindy GymbaROO	www.gymbaroo.com.au
Sensory Integration International	www.sensoryintegration.org.uk
The Learning Breakthrough Program	www.learningbreakthrough.com
Swimming for babies	www.waterbabies.co.uk

2   Sound therapy programmes

ARROW Training	www.self-voice.com
Auditory Integration Training (AIT)	www.AITinstitute.org
Johansen Individual Auditory Stimulation Therapy (JIAST)	www.johansenias.com
Musica Medica	www.musicamedica.ch
The Listening Fitness Program (Lift)	www.listeningfitness.com
The Listening Program (Doman)	www.thelisteningprogram.com
SONATAL (pre-natal to age seven)	www.sonatal.ru

3   Music education

The Voice Foundation	www.voicefoundation.org
Dalcroze (music education with the body)	www.dalcroze.org.uk
Choir Schools Association	www.choirschools.org.uk

4   Sensory training

Association for Infant Massage	www.iaim.org.uk

5   Organizations providing information, advice and support

Dyspraxia Foundation	www.dyspraxiafoundation.org.uk
Dyslexia Action	www.dyslexiaaction.org.uk
Hyperactive Children's Support Group	www.hacsg.org.uk

ICan – charity supporting children's speech and language development　www.ican.org.uk

Association For All Speech Impaired Children (AFASIC)　www.afasic.org.uk

Infant mental health/autism　www.infantmentalhealth.com

6　Nutritional Screening (non-medical)

Foresight – charity for pre-conceptual care　www.foresight-preconception.org.uk

Other books by Sally Goddard Blythe

Reflexes, Learning and Behaviour. Fern Ridge Press. Eugene 2002. Revised 2005.

The Well Balanced Child. Hawthorn Press, Stroud 2004.

What Babies and Children Really Need. Hawthorn Press, Stroud 2008.

Attention, Balance and Coordination – the A,B,C of Learning Success. Wiley, Chichester 2009.

Assessing neuro-motor readiness for learning. The INPP developmental screening test and school intervention programme. Due to be published autumn 2011 by Wiley-Blackwell. Chichester.

Bibliography

American Associates, Ben-Gurion University of the Negev. 'Hand-clapping songs improve motor and cognitive skills, research shows.' Science Daily. 3/5/2010. wwww.sciencedaily.com/releases.2010/04/100428090954. htm Rowe N. 1996. Personal communication.

Barsch R.H., 1968. *Achieving Perceptual-Motor Efficiency. A Space Oriented Approach to Learning. Volume 1 of a perceptual-motor curriculum.* Special Child Publications. Seattle.WA.

Berthoz A., 2000. *The Brain's Sense of Movement.* Harvard University Press, Cambridge.

Bortlle J.E., 2001. 'The Bortle Dark-Sky Scale.' Sky & Telescope. http://www.skyandtelescope.com/resources/darksky/3304011.html. Retrieved 2009-11-18

Boyatzis C., Chazan E., Ting C.Z., 1993. 'Preschool children's decoding of facial emotions.' *Journal of Genetic Psychology,* 154: 375–82.

Capute A.J., Accardo P.J., 1991. *Developmental Disabilities in Infancy and Childhood.* Paul Brookes Publishing Company, Baltimore.

Caramazza A., Journal reference: Proceedings of the National Academics of Science (DOI: 10.1073/pnas.0902262106). Cited in: P Shetty. 'Role of the mirror neurons may need a rethink.' *New Scientist Life.* 27/10. May 2009.

Coward R., 2009. 'Is modern society bad for children?' – Debate at Roehampton University http://www.theinstituteofwellbeing.com/blog/?p=433&cpage=1.

Darwin C., 1872. *The Expression of Emotions in Animals.* John Murray, London.

Durden-Smith J., de Simone D., 1983. *Sex and the Brain.* Pan Books Ltd., London.

Early childhood education and care in Finland. Brochures of the Ministry of Social Affairs and Health 2004: 14.

Eckerdal P., Merker B. 'Music and the action song in infant development: An interpretation.' Cited in: Colwyn Trevarthen and Stephen Malloch (eds), 2009. *Communicative Musicality. Exploring the Basis of Human Companionship.* Oxford University Press.

Eliot L., 2009. *Pink Brain, Blue Brain. How Small Differences Grow into Troublesome Gaps – and what we can do about it.* Hougton Mifflin Harcourt, New York.

'For comfort, mom's voice works as well as a hug.' ScienceDaily.com. Science News www.sciencedaily.com. 12 May, 2010.

Gallese V., Fadiga I. and Rizzolatti G., 1996. 'Action recognition in the pre-motor cortex.' *Brain* 119: 593–609.

Gibran K., 1982. *The Prophet.* Heineman, London.

Goddard Blythe S.A., 2008. *What Babies and Children Really Need.* Hawthorn Press, Stroud.

Goddard Blythe S.A., 1996. Revised 2007. *The INPP Test Battery and Developmental Movement Programme for use in Schools with Children with Special Educational Needs.* Restricted Publication. INPP Chester.

Goddard Blythe S.A., 2003. *The Well Balanced Child.* Hawthorn Press, Stroud.

Goddard Blythe S.A., 2005. 'Releasing educational potential through movement. A summary of individual studies carried out using The INPP test battery and developmental exercise programme for use in schools with special needs.' *Child Care in Practice.* 11/4: 415–32.

Goddard Blythe S.A., 2008. *What Babies and Children Really Need.* Hawthorn Press, Stroud.

Goddard Blythe S.A., 2010. 'Why boys and girls have different needs in the early years.' *Montessori International.*95: 14–18.

Gross J., 2009. Cited in article: 'End of bedtime stories is wrecking children's speech warns government's new "communications champion".' Laura Clark. Daily Mail, 16 October 2009.

Gross J., 2010. Cited in article: 'Middle class parents too busy to teach their children how to talk says "communications champion".' Laura Clark. Daily Mail, 1 January 2010.

Haeckel E., 1899. *Riddle of the Universe at the Close of the Nineteenth Century.*

Halleck R.P., 1898. *The Education of the Nervous System.* The Macmillan Company, New York.

Harlow H.F., 1958. 'The Nature of Love', *American Psychologist*, 13, 573–685

House R., 2009. 'Is modern society bad for children?' – Debate at Roehampton University

http://www.theinstituteofwellbeing.com/blog/?p=433 &cpage=1

http://www.famousquotes.me.uk/nursery_rhymes/hey_diddle_diddle.htm

http://www.howkidsdevelop.com/developDevDelay.html

http://www.hymnsandcarolsofchristmas.com/Hymns_and_Carols/rocking_carol-2.htm

http://www.lizlyle.lofgrens.org/RmOlSngs/RTOS-CoventryCarol.html

Kiphard E.J., 1980. 'Psychiatrist clown relieves children's fears.' Article received via personal communication. Provenance unknown.

Kiphard E.J., 2000. 'Intervention programmes using the German psycho-motor approach with exceptional children.' Paper presented at The 12th European Conference of Neuro-Developmental Delay in Children with Specific Learning Difficulties. Chester, March 2000.

Kraus N., 2010. 'Cognitive sensory interaction in the neural encoding of speech and music.' Paper presented at Symposium on: Music-Language Interactions in the Brain: From the Brainstem to Broca's Area. Presentation to The American Association for the Advancement of Science Conference. February 2010.

Labarthe J.C., 1997. 'Are boys better than girls at building a tower or a bridge at 2 years of age?' *Archives of Diseases of Childhood*. 77: 140–4.

Lane C., http://www.self-voice.com

Lazarev M., 2007. *Mammababy: Birth Before Birth*. Olma Media Group, Moscow.

Meltzoff A.N., Moore M.K., 1977. 'Imitation of facial and manual gestures by human neonates.' *Science* 198: 75–8.

Meltzoff A.N., Moore M.K., 1983. 'Newborn infants imitate adults facial gestures.' *Child Development*. 54: 702–9.

Milne A.A., 1927. *Now We Are Six*. Methuen and Company, London.

Mines S., 'I Can Feel My Baby Move! Prenatal Developmental Movement and Parental Response.' http://www.selfgrowth.com/articles/Mines1.html http://www.babyhut.co.uk/

Norfleet James A., 2007. *Teaching the Male Brain*. Corwin Press, CA.

Panksepp J., 1998. *Affective Neuroscience. The Foundations of Human and Animal Emotions*. Oxford University Press, New York.

Panksepp J., 2007. 'Can play diminish ADHD and facilitate the construction of the social brain?' *J Can Acad Child Adolesc Psychiatry*. 16/2: 57–66.

Patel A.D., Burnham E.J., 2010. 'Music, language and grammatical processing.' Paper presented at Symposium on: Music-Language Interactions in the Brain: From the Brainstem to Broca's Area. Presentation to The American Association for the Advancement of Science Conference. New York

Schiftan Y., 2009. *The Missing Link. Musica Medica – Good vibrations. A new method of multisensory brain & body stimulation*. Unpublished manuscript. Reproduced by permission of the author.

Schore A., 1994. *Affect Regulation and the Origin of the Self*. Laurence Erlbaum, Hove.

Schrager O., 2000. 'Balance control, age and language development.' Paper presented at The 12th European Conference of Neuro-Developmental Delay in Children with Specific Learning Difficulties. Chester, March 2000.

Shaywitz S.E., 1996. *Dyslexia*. Scientific American. November pp.77–104.

Small M.F., 1999. *Our Babies Ourselves. How biology and culture shape the way we parent*. Anchor Books.

Steindl-Rast D., 1995. *The Music of Silence*. Harper, San Francisco

Stocks M., Maddocks A., 1992. *Growing with Music. Key stage 1 Teacher's book*. Longman Group UK.

Storr A., 1993, *Music and the Mind*. Harper Collins, London

Stratford T., Mera A., 2009. 'The neurobiology of the therapeutic relationship between client and therapist: targeting symptomatic anxiety.' The 10th NPSA Congress. Paris, 20 June 2009.

Suite101: 'Medieval Christmas Carols pt. 1: Origins' http://medievalhistory. suite101.com/article.cfm/medieval_christmas_carols_pt__1# ixzz0gv8Q8B3C

Taylor J., Taylor A., 1806. *Rhymes for the Nursery*.

The NIH/NIMH study. 2007. 'Sexual dimorphism of brain developmental trajectories during childhood and adolescence.' *NeuroImage*.36/4: 165–73.

Thompson T., undated. Cited in article 'Say Goodnight to Sleepless Nights with Lullabies' by Sarah Molnar. http://www.curiousparents.

Trevarthen C., 2007. 'To be conscious: How infants' movements are planned, and how they engage with stimuli, things and people.' Paper presented at The 18th European Conference of Neuro-Developmental Delay in Children with Specific Learning Difficulties. Pisa, September 23 2007.

Zeedyk, S., 2008. Cited in: Curtis, P: 'Type of buggy can affect baby development, study finds.' *The Guardian* 21.11.2008.

Zeedyk S, 2008. 'Talk to your baby.' Baby buggies may undermine child development. National Literacy Trust, 21.11.2008

Index

CREATIVE, INSPIRING AND PRACTICAL BOOKS FOR THRIVING CHILDREN

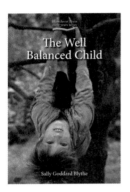

The Well Balanced Child
Movement and early learning
SALLY GODDARD BLYTHE

'Learning is not just about reading, writing and maths,' says Sally Goddard Blythe. 'A child's experience of movement will help play a pivotal role in shaping his personality, his feelings and achievements.' Her book makes the case for a 'whole body' approach to learning which integrates the brain, senses, movement, music and play. *The Well Balanced Child* examines why movement matters; how music helps brain development; the role of nutrition, the brain and child growth; and offers practical tips for parents and educators to help children with learning and behavioural problems.

'... *compelling and enthusiastic. A strong book with important messages about early years learning.*' The Teacher

240pp; 216 × 138mm; 978-1-903458-63-1; pb; **£12.99**

What Babies and Children Really Need
How mothers and fathers can nurture children's growth for health and wellbeing
SALLY GODDARD BLYTHE

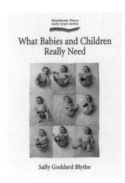

This book represents a milestone in our understanding of child development and what parents can do to give their children the best start in life. *What Babies Really Need* draws on the latest scientific research to show how a baby's relationship with its mother has a lasting and fundamental impact. Sally Goddard Blythe calls for a new Charter for Childhood in which nutrition, play, affection and discipline are valued as the basic building blocks for meeting children's needs.

'*This comprehensive book provides parents with the information they need to raise healthy, balanced, resilient children ... Above all, it demonstrates that what babies really need is the time, love and attention of the loving adults in their lives.*'
Sue Palmer, author of *Toxic Childhood*

368pp; 234 × 156mm; 978-1-903458-76-1; pb; **£16.99**

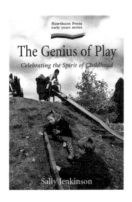

The Genius of Play
Celebrating the spirit of childhood
SALLY JENKINSON

Imagine a teaching aid which enhanced a child's self esteem and social skills, enriched their imagination, and encouraged creative thinking. That teaching aid is play. Sally Jenkinson argues that even as a growing body of research helps us to understand the genius of play we are eroding children's self-initiated play with inappropriate toys, TV and consumerism.

'... *a book of genius, which celebrates childhood magically and enchantingly by capturing its spirit throughout ...*'
Diane Rich, *Early Education*

224pp; 216 × 138mm; 978-1-903458-04-4; pb; **£12.99**

CREATIVE, INSPIRING AND PRACTICAL BOOKS FOR THRIVING CHILDREN

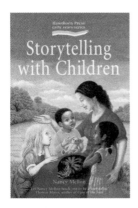

Storytelling with Children
NANCY MELLON

Telling stories is a peaceful, magical way of creating special occasions with children, whether it is at bedtime, around the fire or on rainy days. Nancy Mellon shows how you can become a confident storyteller with a wealth of ideas for using stories with dance, rhyme, puppets and creative play.

'Nancy Mellon's experience, advice and suggestions work wonders. They are potent seeds that give you the creative confidence to find your own style of storytelling.'
Ashley Ramsden, Director of the School of Storytelling, Emerson College

192pp; 216 × 138mm; 978-1-903458-08-2; pb; **£9.99**

Healing Stories for Challenging Behaviour
SUSAN PERROW

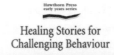

Healing Stories for
Challenging Behaviour

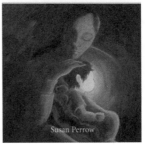

Susan Perrow writes, collects and documents stories that offer a therapeutic journey for the listener – a positive, imaginative way of healing difficult situations. Her collection of modern and traditional folk stories includes stories for challenging behaviours such as dishonesty, stealing, bullying and fighting; and stories for challenging situations such as moving house, a new baby, nightmares, illness or grieving. Each story is introduced with notes and suggestions for use. There is also a guide to help readers create their own healing stories.

'Explore the ancient art of storytelling with this inspiring book, strengthening your connection with your child along the way.' Kindred Magazine

320pp; 234 × 156mm; 978-1-903458-78-5; pb; **£14.99**

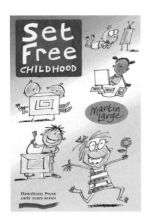

Set Free Childhood
Parents' survival guide to coping with computers and TV
MARTIN LARGE

Children watch TV and use computers for five hours daily on average. The result? Record levels of learning difficulties, obesity, eating disorders, sleep problems, language delay, aggressive behaviour, anxiety – and children on fast forward. *Set Free Childhood* shows you how to counter screen culture and create a calmer, more enjoyable family life.

'His practical suggestions empower readers to take charge of their children's upbringing and make it essential reading for all parents. I urge you to read this important book.' Five to El'

240pp; 216 × 138mm; 978-1-903458-43-3; pb; **£10.99**

CREATIVE, INSPIRING AND PRACTICAL BOOKS FOR THRIVING CHILDREN

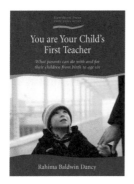

You Are Your Child's First Teacher
What parents can do with and for their children from birth to age six
RAHIMA BALDWIN DANCY

This lucid, practical and common-sense guide will help you navigate safely through the early years of childhood and find solutions that work for your own family situation. Create your own family rituals to ease the daily routine, nourish your child's imagination with simple, home-made toys and materials from the garden and kitchen cupboard, and use imitation, repetition and setting limits to promote a harmonious family life.

'One of the most readable and accessible books on parenting... Rahima shows a way of understanding child development that encourages respect and love for the natural unfolding of emotional life, intelligence and creativity in the young child.'
Kindling

400pp; 234 × 156mm; 978-1-903458-65-5; pb; **£14.99**

Free to Learn
Introducing Steiner Waldorf early childhood education
LYNNE OLDFIELD

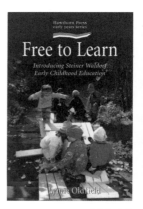

Free to Learn is a comprehensive introduction to Steiner Waldorf kindergartens for parents, educators and early years' students. It draws on the theory and practice of kindergarten education around the world with stories, helpful insights and lively observations. Author Lynne Oldfield is Director of the London Waldorf Early Childhood Teacher Training Course.

'... a timely contribution to the debate about appropriate early education and a balanced approach to what, when and how children learn.'
Nursery World

256pp; 216 × 138mm; 978-1-903458-06-8; pb; **£11.99**

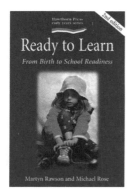

Ready to Learn (2nd edition)
From birth to school readiness
MARTYN RAWSON AND MICHAEL ROSE

Ready to Learn will help you to decide when your child is ready to take the step from kindergarten to school proper. The key is an imaginative grasp of how children learn to play, speak, think and relate between birth and six years of age.

'Sound points about the risks of making developmentally inappropriate demands, including the headlong rush to get children to read and write ever earlier.' Jennie Lindon, *Nursery World*

224pp; 216 × 138mm; 978-1-903458-66-2; pb; **£10.99**